GESTODENE

GESTODENE
Development of a new gestodene-containing low-dose oral contraceptive

*The Proceedings of a Special Satellite Symposium held
in conjunction with the XIth World Congress
of Gynecology and Obstetrics*

Edited by Max Elstein

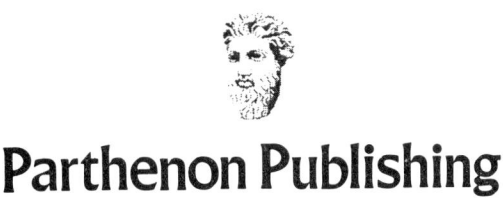

Parthenon Publishing
THE PARTHENON PUBLISHING GROUP LIMITED

Company Note

The monophasic preparation of 75 μg gestodene combined with 30 μg ethinyl estradiol will be marketed under the following brand names:

Femodene®, Gynera®, Femovan® and Ginoden®

These names are all registered trade marks of Schering AG, West Germany.

The views expressed in the text are those of the participants and do not necessarily represent those of Schering AG, West Germany.

Published in the UK and Europe by
The Parthenon Publishing Group Limited,
Casterton Hall, Carnforth,
Lancs. LA6 2LA, England   ISBN 1–85070–100–8

Printed in Great Britain

Contents

List of contributors

S. Beier
Fachgebiet weibliche Fertilitätsforschung
und experimentelle Gynäkologie
Schering Aktiengesellschaft
Müllerstr. 170–178
1000 Berlin 65
Germany

P. Bye
Schering Health-Care
The Brow
Burgess Hill
West Sussex RH15 9NE
Great Britain

B. Cesana
Clinica Medica I
Università degli Studi di Milano
Via F. Forza 35
20122 Milano
Italy

E. N. Chantler
Senior Lecturer in Reproductive Biochemistry
Withington Hospital
Department of Obstetrics and Gynaecology
Nell Lane, West Didsbury
Manchester M20 8LR
Great Britain

P. G. Crosignani
Clinica Ostetrica e Ginecologica III
Università degli Studi di Milano
Via M. Melloni 52
20129 Milano
Italy

B. Düsterberg
Segment Endokrinotherapie und
Fertilitätskontrolle
Schering Aktiengesellschaft
Müllerstr. 170–178
1000 Berlin 65
Germany

W. Elger
Leiter des Fachgebietes weibliche
Fertilitätsforschung und experimentelle
Gynäkologie
Schering Aktiengesellschaft
Müllerstr. 170–178
1000 Berlin 65
Germany

M. Elstein
Professor of Obstetrics and Gynaecology
University Hospital of South Manchester
Department of Obstetrics and
Gynaecology
Nell Lane, West Didsbury
Manchester M20 8LR
Great Britain

E. Eyong
University Hospital of South Manchester
Department of Obstetrics and
Gynaecology
Nell Lane, West Didsbury
Manchester M20 8LR
Great Britain

F. Franceschetti
Laboratorio del Servizio di Fislopatologia
della Riproduzione Umana
Università degli Studi di Bologna
Via Massarenti 13
40138 Bologna
Italy

G. Giudici
Cattedra Semelotica Medica
Università degli Studi di Milano
Via Pace 9
20122 Milano
Italy

N. Y. Haboubi
Department of Histopathology
Withington Hospital
Nell Lane, West Didsbury
Manchester M20 8LR
Great Britain

H. Hannse
Mitglied des Vorstandes der
Schering Aktiengesellschaft
Müllerstr. 170–178
1000 Berlin 65
Germany

M. Hümpel
Leiter des Hauptdepartments
Pharmacokinetik
Schering Aktiengesellschaft
Müllerstr. 170–178
1000 Berlin 65
Germany

R. J. Kirkman
Principal Medical Officer
Central Health Clinic
1 Mulberry Street
Sheffield S1 2PJ
Great Britain

W. Krause
Leiter des Departments Pharmacokinetik B
Schering Aktiengesellschaft
Müllerstr. 170–178
1000 Berlin 65
Germany

H. Kuhl
Abteilung für Gynäkologie
Endokrinologie
Zentrum der Frauenheilkunde und
Geburtshilfe
Johann-Wolfgang-Goethe-Universität
Theodor-Stern-Kai 7
6000 Frankfurt
Germany

U. Lachnit-Fixson
Leiterin des Fachbereichs Klinische
Forschung
Schering Aktiengesellschaft
Müllerstr. 170–178
1000 Berlin 65
Germany

W. Losert
Leiter des Fachgebietes
Allgemeine Pharmakologie
Schering Aktiengesellschaft
Müllerstr. 170–178
1000 Berlin 65
Germany

R. Orlandi
Medical Department of
Schering SpA
Via Cassanese
20090 Segrate Milano
Italy

B. Runnebaum
Ärztlicher Direktor
Abteilung für Gynäkologische
Endokrinologie
Universitäts-Frauenklinik
Voss Str. 9
6900 Heidelberg 1
Germany

E. Schillinger
Leiter des Fachgebietes
Biochemische Pharmakologie
Schering Aktiengesellschaft
Müllerstr. 170–178
1000 Berlin 65
Germany

R. Sharma
University Hospital of South Manchester
Department of Obstetrics
and Gynaecology
Nell Lane, West Didsbury
Manchester M20 8LR
Great Britain

J. Spona
Leiter der Abteilung für
Experimentelle Endokrinologie
und Humanlaboratorium
1. Universitäts-Frauenklinik
Spitalgasse 23
1090 Vienna
Austria

H. Steinbeck
Former staff member in
the main department of
Endocrine Pharmacology
Schering Aktiengesellschaft
Müllerstr. 170–178
1000 Berlin 65
Germany

J. W. Tack
Leiter des Departments Galenik
Schering Aktiengesellschaft
Müllerstr. 170–178
1000 Berlin 65
Germany

R. Unger
Klinische Forschung
Schering Aktiengesellschaft
Müllerstr. 170–178
1000 Berlin 65
Germany

F. Vergadoro
Clinica Ostetrica e Ginecologica III
Universita degli Studi di Milano
Via M. Melloni 52
20129 Milano
Italy

G. Vergani
Cattedra Semelotica Medica
Università degli Studi di Milano
Via Pace 9
20122 Milano
Italy

G. Vigotti
Cattedra Semelotica Medica
Università degli Studi di Milano
Via F. Forza 35
20122 Milano
Italy

Foreword

M. Elstein

In the quarter of a century since oral contraceptives were introduced in Europe there have been major advances. These have been made possible by knowledge gained from extensive clinical experience, decreasing the dosage resulting in improved formulations and novel and more selective compounds. These contraceptive products have therefore become more acceptable with reduced side-effects. Additionally with these improvements, the evidence suggests that the products have less adverse effects. This has vindicated the policy of minimal dosage for desired action yet maintaining effectiveness and acceptability.

The association between thromboembolism and estrogen generated an approach to reduce the dosage of estrogen to $30\,\mu$g and this was facilitated by the synthesis of the 18 homologated 19 nor-steroid, levonorgestrel by Hershel Smith and finally the elimination of its inactive enantiomer. This progestogen has enabled the development of combined products with a significant decrease in total steroid dose and good acceptor compliance because of the low incidence of side-effects. A further improvement was the triphasic concept with a further reduction in progestogen dosage which became even more relevant when cardiovascular adverse effects seemed to be related to the dosage of progestogen.

This publication describes the scientific basis and early clinical experience of a low-estrogen combined formulation with a lower dose of a new progestogen, Gestodene. This progestogen, by the introduction of a $\varDelta^{15}$ double bond, has shown evidence of greater inhibition of pituitary-ovarian function and a more profound genital tract effect than levonorgestrel. This enhanced endocrinal activity has been achieved without undesirable metabolic effects. Hence in the dosage used in the combined estrogen-progestogen formulation there is considerable advance in reaching the objective of an oral contraceptive which has further minimized adverse effects and yet achieves effective contraception with good acceptability.

Ongoing studies in the development of the new progestogen Gestodene are described. Many of these data, which were presented at the Satellite symposium on the occasion of the 11th World Congress of Gynecology and Obstetrics, Berlin, in September 1985 have been extended, and indeed completed, and are now included in this volume.

Preface

H. Hannse

We should like to introduce you to an extremely low-dosage contraceptive which was created on the basis of a new progestogen developed in our laboratories. It is anticipated that it will be licensed for use by the Federal Health Authority in the near future.* Its introduction in the Federal Republic of Germany will coincide with the 25th jubilee of the introduction of the preparation Anovlar®, with which we initiated the era of hormonal contraception in Europe. Allow me on this occasion to look back on the contributions made by Schering research which permitted the realization of the principle of contraception by the inhibition of ovulation.

We are indebted to the American Dr Gregory Pincus and co-workers for practical trials with estrogen-progestogen combinations. The most important preconditions for the development of preparations of this type were established by Schering research in the 1930s. In 1932, Hohlweg and Junkmann published their findings on the control of the functions of the anterior lobe of the pituitary gland by the diencephalon which were discovered in Schering's main laboratory. They were the first to recognize the cybernetic mechanism of regulation in the triangle consisting of the hypothalamus, the pituitary gland and the gonads, which was the initial prerequisite to develop the mechanism of the inhibition of ovulation by estrogen-progestogen combinations.

The same year Butenandt succeeded in elucidating the structure of a natural estrogen, estrone, which had already been isolated in cooperation with Schering in 1929.

This was followed in 1934 by identification of the pure natural corpus luteum hormone, progesterone, and elucidation of its structure. Economical synthesis of these two hormones, starting from cholesterol, was likewise developed at Schering, as well as the synthesis of the strongest natural estrogen, estradiol, by hydration of estrone in 1933, two years before it was isolated from natural material.

The disadvantage of these steroid hormones was that they remained practically ineffective when administered orally. The decisive breakthrough involved the synthesis of the first orally effective sex hormones, namely ethinyl estradiol and ethisterone, by Inhoffen in 1938; ethinyl

* Approval dated from January 1987 has been received.

estradiol is still the most widely used estrogen component of all ovulation inhibitors in the world and ethisterone is the parent substance for most contraceptive progestogens employed today. After World War II the path led further via norethisterone, first synthesized in 1951 by Djerassi, to norethisterone acetate developed in our house, i.e., the progestogen of our pioneer preparation, Anovlar. Advances in the total synthesis of steroids resulted in 1961 in Hershel Smith producing norgestrel for the first time. This active agent was both qualitatively and quantitatively a considerable improvement. It is a mixture of enantiomers, i.e., two variants of the same molecule differing in the spatial arrangement of the atoms like mirror images of each other. The difficult problem of the synthesis of the only form of this mixture which is biologically active, levonorgestrel, was solved by Schering research by new elegant steps of synthesis. This was made possible by our expertise in biotechnology with the aid of micro-organisms bred specially for this purpose and by new stereo and enantio selective reactions which permit economical production. Levonorgestrel is today the most widely used progestogen employed for hormonal contraception in the world.

After a creative break of almost 10 years our chemists were able to synthesize gestodene in 1975 and we should like to present this substance to you today in the form of a hormonal contraceptive. From the initial synthesis to the anticipated launch a period of approximately 10 years has elapsed. This clearly shows the long and expensive path which must nowadays be trod during product development to arrive at a preparation ready for licensing. More than half of the period of protection provided for by the patent, which in Germany lasts until 1993, has already passed. Further years will pass before its introduction in other important countries, and the still remaining phase of commercial exploitation under protection from imitators will shrink accordingly. This also explains why at present very few firms develop new preparations for fertility control, for the introduction of a new preparation such as we are witnessing today has become a rare occurrence. In future the staff of our pharmaceutical division will be in a position to achieve such successes only if and as long as social politicians leave us an adequate economic basis.

Introduction

B. Runnebaum

Oral hormonal contraceptives belong to the products which have undergone the most intensive testing for desired and unwanted effects. During the past 25 years in which the pill has been in use it has been implicated with a number of serious disorders, principally those concerning the cardiovascular system. Attempts were made to overcome these problems by systematically reducing first the estrogen and then the progestogen dose contained in the pill. On the other hand, as a result of the large prospective studies conducted predominantly in the UK and USA we also became familiar with the advantages to health which are associated with taking the pill. In recent years there have been repeated discussions and reports on its advantages and disadvantages. Thus, after a detailed analysis of contraceptive methods under development, the 1984 symposium in Heidelberg on future aspects in contraception showed that the low-dose pill will remain one of the most important methods of contraception for a long time to come. It is therefore to be welcomed that within the scope of the World Congress of Gynecology and Obstetrics we are still endeavouring today to reduce the frequency of serious side-effects of the pill, or to eliminate them completely, whilst retaining its positive effects. As far as serious complications are concerned, we do not have any statistically relevant figures available as regards the low-dose pill. However, with respect to the high-dose pill containing $50\,\mu g$ and more of ethinyl estradiol and different doses of progestogens, we have gained extensive knowledge from broadly-based prospective studies about the order of magnitude and type of complications occurring with the pill. The mortality figures for pill-takers are fairly reliable and vary between 0 and 20 per 100 000 women-years.

However, as an investigation into the mortality of fertile women in countries with widespread oral contraceptive usage has shown, this estimate is too high. These figures depend on risk factors, race, nutrition and age. Risk factors when taking the pill include smoking, obesity, diabetus mellitus and hypertension as well as cardiovascular diseases. The role that these factors, cardiovascular diseases and the hormone doses in the pill play is largely unknown.

As regards morbidity, assessment becomes more difficult, since in addition to registration of risk factors, environmental influences and nutrition there is the problem of validating the diagnosis of a certain disease. In the case of morbidity, it is primarily the serious, i.e., life-threatening complications that are of interest. They are rare but could increasingly occur in apparently healthy women who take the pill as was shown by epidemiological studies with higher dosed preparations.

If it were possible to eliminate the cardiovascular problems under discussion in healthy women by prescribing the low-dose pill (30–35μg ethinyl estradiol and a suitable low-dose progestogen), then the advantages of the pill would clearly become more apparent.

Table 1 shows the pill's advantages and disadvantages. The definitive advantages, apart from high contraceptive reliability and reversibility of the method, are reliable cycle control and regular menstruation, as well as distinctly increased protection from pelvic inflammation and some neoplastic diseases. A problem that still has to be resolved is the prevention of cardiovascular complications. Many advantages of the pill are clearly dependent on the progestogen. The low estrogen dose is sufficient for cycle control and reliably prevents osteoporosis over the years of using the pill. The estrogen dose of 30 μg of ethinyl estradiol can be reduced only if certain delivery systems guarantee uniform estrogen levels over 24-hour periods. As a function

Table 1   Advantages and disadvantages of the pill

Advantages	*Disadvantages*
1. High contraceptive reliability	1. To be taken daily
2. Method is reversible	2. Difficult to keep secret
3. No disturbance of privacy and coitus	3. Negative (i.e., injurious) effects from
4. Positive (i.e., beneficial) effects on:	epidemiological studies on:
– dysfunctional bleeding	– cardiovascular system
– iron deficiency anemia	– myocardial infarction
– premenstrual syndrome	– thromboembolism
– dysmenorrhea	– cerebral hemorrhage
– acne, seborrhea, hirsutism	– thrombosis
– myomas	– hypertension
– endometriosis	– metabolic disturbances
– rheumatoid arthritis	– liver tumors
5. Distinct protection from:	
– ovarian cysts	
– benign breast tumours	
– ovarian cancer	
– endometrial cancer	
– salpingitis, tubal pregnancy	

of dose, estrogens are primarily responsible for venous thrombosis, and progestogens probably for thromboembolism in the arterial system.

According to C.R. Kay* the incidence of arterial disease seems to increase under higher progestogen dosages but not when the estrogen dose is being raised. Type and dose of the progestogen used seem to influence the blood pressure as can be seen in Figure 1.

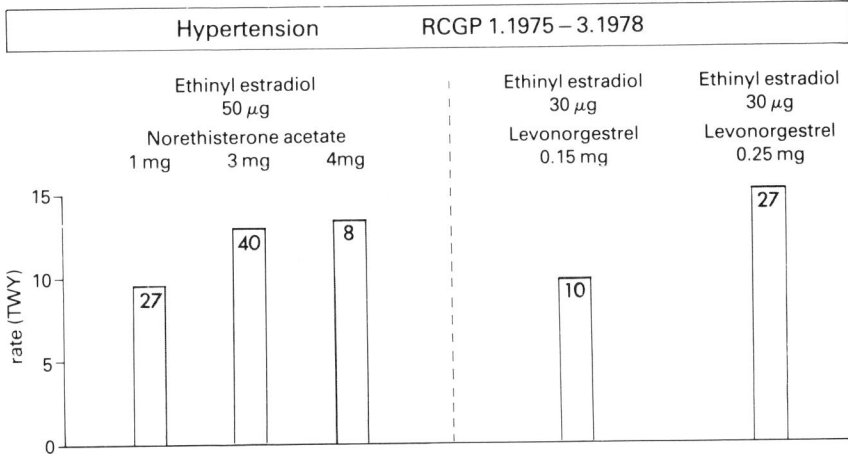

Figure 1

At this point in time, the following statements can be made and questions raised regarding the pill:

1. The low-dose pill is the ideal contraceptive method for young women and shows considerable advantages to their health. The cardiovascular risk associated with the pill is low under the low-dose pill, but cannot be substantiated by epidemiological data as yet.
2. It is unclear why the progestogens have a negative influence on the blood vessels. It is assumed that some progestogens at certain concentrations show unfavourable effects on lipid, glucose, insulin, renin and angiotensin levels thereby affecting the cardiovascular system. It is our challenge for the future to establish which progestogen at which dose does not show any negative effect on the metabolism and the cardiovascular system. Schering scientists such

*RCGP – study.

as Dr. Hofmeister, Dr. Laurent and Prof. Wiechert have developed a new progestogen, gestodene. This substance shows new effects from a qualitative and quantitative point of view. We will today hear important reports on this new pill containing gestodene, a pill with the lowest ever progestogen content.

1

Endocrine-pharmacological profile of gestodene

W. Elger, H. Steinbeck, E. Schillinger, W. Losert and S. Beier

Since the introduction of the first hormonal contraceptives the tolerance of these products has been a major consideration in their subsequent development.

Substances were introduced into the therapy, such as levonorgestrel, for example, which permitted very much lower doses of the progestogen component than had been possible with any of the previously known progestogens, and which were also able to balance excessive and undesirable effects of the estrogen component in these oral contraceptives. The anti-androgen cyproterone acetate proved to be a welcome addition to this form of therapy as its inclusion in oral contraceptives elicited effective management of androgenization symp-

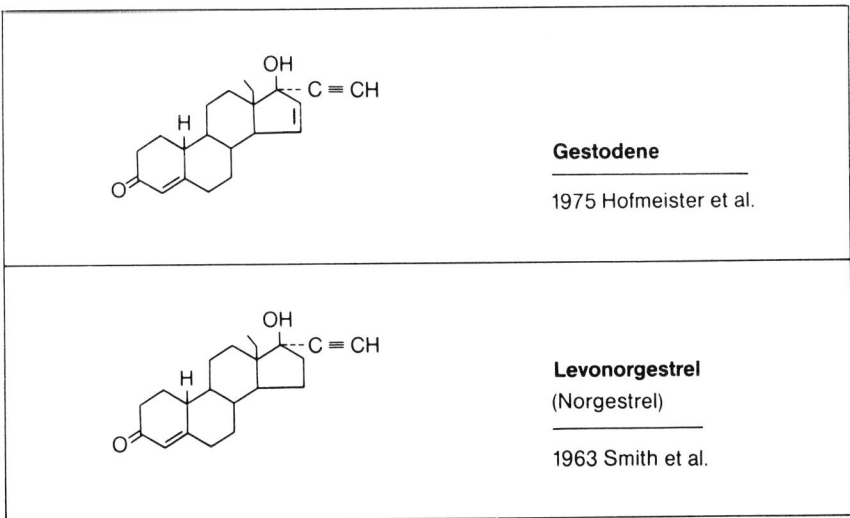

Figure 1   Structural formulae

toms of the skin in oral contraceptive users in addition to its contraceptive efficacy[1,2].

It must not be forgotten, however, that dose reduction and the fitting
of the therapy to the course of the estrogen and progesterone levels in
the normal cycle contributed just as much to the high standard of
modern hormonal contraception[3].

The development of gestodene[4,5] has made a further substance
from the 19-nortestosterone series available for clinical use in oral
contraceptives. Its activity and hormonal profile set new standards
(Figure 1).

In terms of present-day understanding, the profile of an oral contraceptive is not represented by the sum of the effects of its estrogen
and progestogen components, but by complex interaction between the
two. This applies both to their influence on sexual functions and to
their effect on the metabolism[6] (Figure 2).

This interaction can be manifested in powerful synergism in the
sexual functions, but can also be expressed in reciprocal negation of
action. In this context, the ability of a progestogen to neutralize
excessive estrogenic effects is of particular relevance as far as hepatic
effects are concerned (Figure 3).

The current state of our knowledge of this aspect indicates that
several properties of the progestogen play an important part here.
These include its progestogenic, estrogenic, androgenic, anti-estrogenic and anti-mineralocorticoid properties.

BINDING PROPERTIES OF GESTODENE TO VARIOUS RECEPTORS AND TRANSPORT PROTEINS

Gestodene exhibits differing degrees of affinity for the various binding
sites for steroid hormones[7]. It binds with high affinity at the progesterone receptor and also has affinity for the androgen, cortisol and
aldosterone receptors, in addition to the sex-hormone-binding globulin
(SHBG). Its relatively powerful affinity for the aldosterone receptor was
very obvious. There was no affinity for the estrogen receptors. The
pattern of binding at the hormone receptor is qualitatively very similar
to that of progesterone, which is in no way confined to the progesterone
receptor (Table 1).

PRECLINICAL INVESTIGATIONS WITH GESTODENE

The following report describes the most pertinent characteristics of
gestodene identified in animal studies. Most of the data were obtained
in tests using parenteral, i.e., subcutaneous injection. It is well known
that most substances of the 19-nortestosterone series exhibit poor

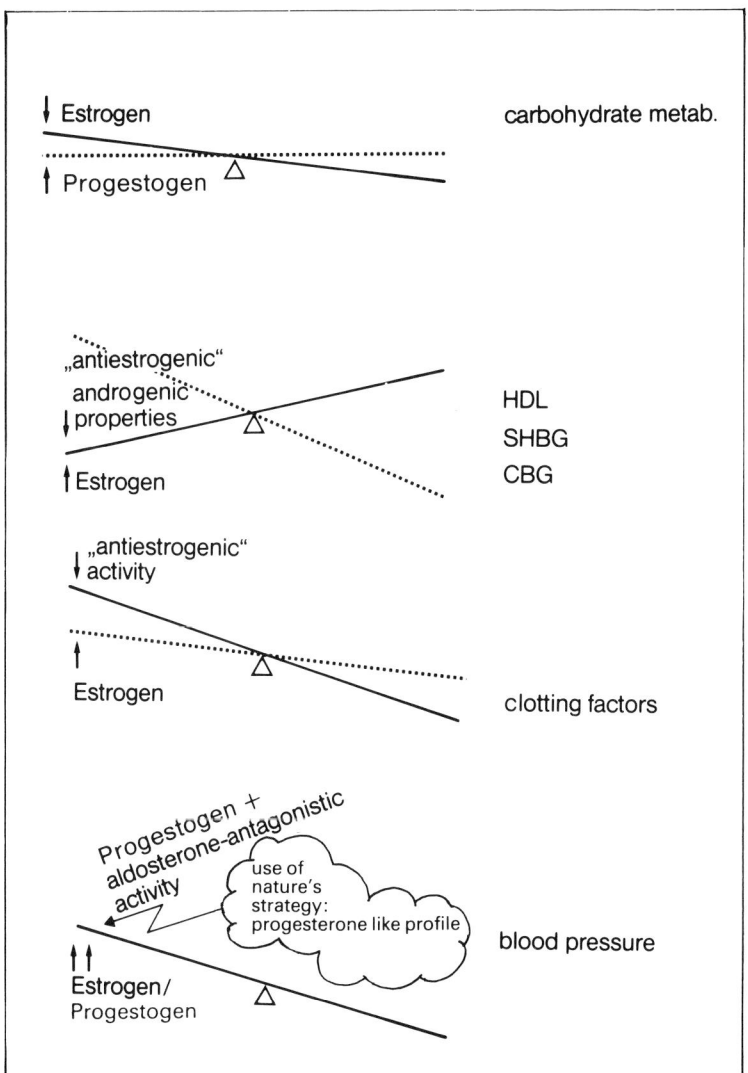

Figure 2   Interaction of progestogen and estrogen at the level of some metabolic effects of oral contraceptives (schematic)

bioavailability in most laboratory animals when given orally and that they circulate in the blood for too short a period to be able to display their inherent activity to the full. Conversely, our use of a formulation in oily solution given by parenteral administration elicits pharmacokinetic and pharmacodynamic behaviour which could be indicative of the effects in man following oral administration[8].

Table 1   Relative binding affinities (RBA) of various progestogens to different receptor sites and transport proteins[7]

Steroid	RBA-values (in %)						
	Prog.-Rec. ^{3}H-R5020	Gluc.-Rec. ^{3}H-Dex.	Min.-Rec. ^{3}H-Ald.	Estradiol-Rec. ^{3}H-E$_2$	Androgen-Rec. ^{3}H-R1881[*]	SHBG ^{3}H-DHT	CBG ^{3}H-Cortisol
Gestodene	85	27	350	< 0.01	90	40	< 0.01
Levonorgestrel	150	< 0.1	120	< 0.01	n.t.	12.5 (50)	< 0.01
Progesterone	50	10	110	< 0.1	< 0.01	< 0.1	30

Dex. = Dexamethasone; Ald. = Aldosterone; E$_2$ = Estradiol; DHT = Dihydrotestosterone

n.t. = not tested; ( ) = repeated test

Pollow et al., unpublished data (1983/84)
[*] Competition factor with [3]H-5α-DHT, rat prostate: Gestodene 1.6, Levonorgestrel 2.0
   (Schillinger et al., Dept. of Biochemical Pharmacology/Schering AG)

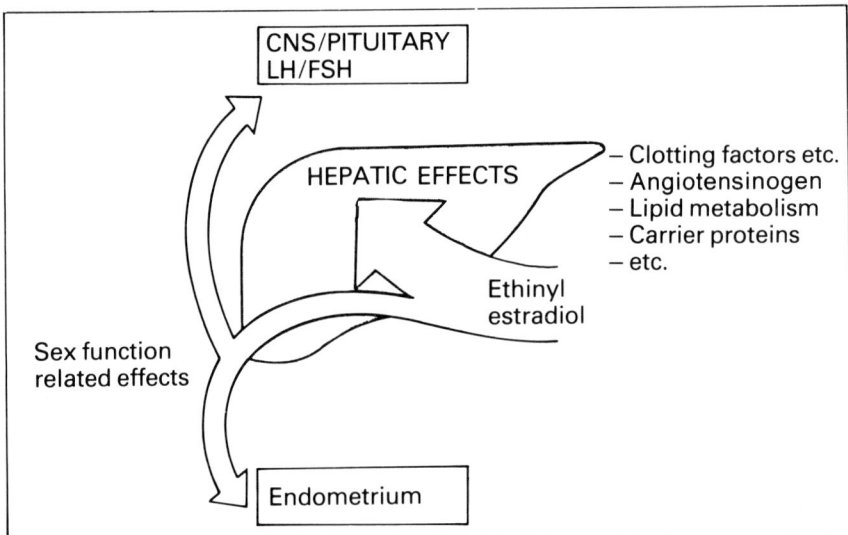

Figure 3   Problem of metabolic estrogen effects. Also marginal doses which control endometrial function (30 μg ethinyl estradiol/day) elevate estrogen-dependent hepatic functions above normal level in women. Some progestogens in part counteract or even reverse some of these effects

Progestogenic and anti-gonadotropic effects

The Clauberg test is the standard method of determining pro-gestogenic activity, as it detects the capacity of the progestogen to transform the estrogen-stimulated endometrium (Figure 4). The right-

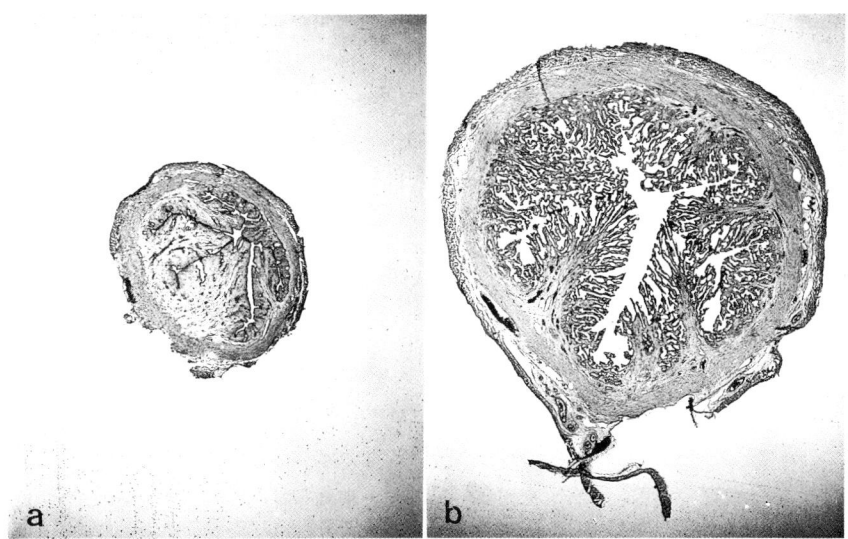

Figure 4   Gestodene-induced endometrial transformation in an estrogen-primed infantile rabbit. Total gestodene dose: 30 μg s.c. (b); estrogen-treated control (a)

hand portion of Figure 4 shows this classic reaction. As far as this reaction is concerned, gestodene is superior to all currently known progestogens (Figure 5).

When administered subcutaneously in the Clauberg test gestodene is active in a total dose of $10-30 \mu g$, which means that it is about three times more potent than levonorgestrel (Figure 5). This high progestogenic activity is also evinced in its capacity to maintain pregnancy in spayed gravid rats. We found activity of this kind at a dose of $3-10 \mu g$/animal/day. This is also equivalent to approximately three times more potent activity than levonorgestrel (Figures 5 and 9).

Next to the transformatory effect in the endometrium, inhibition of ovulation is the most important property of a progestogen as far as its use in an oral contraceptive is concerned. Doses of $3 \mu g$ gestodene/day s.c. are adequate for inhibition of ovulation in the rat. This is equivalent to about three to ten times the potency of levonorgestrel (Figure 5).

Progestogen	Dose mg/animal/day	Inhibition of ovulation in rats % s.c.	Maintenance of pregnancy in ovariectomized rats* (♀day 8 – autopsy day 21) % s.c.	Clauberg test in rabbits–endometrial transformation McPhail index ** l)	
				s.c.	p.o.
Gestodene	0.1	–	–	–	3.5 (10)
	0.03	100 (6)	100 (6)	3.1 (9)	2.6 (10)
	0.01	100 (6)	92 (6)	1.8 (10)	1.5 (10)
	0.003	50 (6)	33 (6)	1.0 (9)	1.0 (10)
	0.001	0 (6)	0 (6)	–	–
Levonorgestrel	0.1	–	100 (5)	3.2 (11)	2.3 (10)
	0.03	100 (6)	88 (5)	2.3 (10)	1.1 (8)
	0.01	33 (6)	0 (5)	1.1 (10)	1.0 (11)
	0.003	17 (6)	–	–	–
	0.001	0 (6)	–	–	–
3-Keto-Desogestrel†	0.1	–	88 (6)	–	–
	0.03	100 (6)	58 (6)	–	3.3 (6)
	0.01	100 (6)	57 (6)	–	2.3 (5)
	0.003	33 (6)	0 (6)	–	1.2 (5)
Desogestrel	3.0	–	100 (6)	–	–
	1.0	100 (6)	60 (5)	–	–
	0.3	33 (6)	0 (6)	–	–
	0.1	17 (6)	0 (6)	2.4 (8)	3.3 (5)
	0.03	17 (6)	0 (6)	1.2 (8)	2.8 (6)
	0.01	–	–	1.0 (7)	1.4 (8)

Figure 5   Evaluation of the progestogenic activity of various progestogens in rats and rabbits

( ) = number of treated animals/groups: – = not tested
* = progestogen was administered together with 1.0 μg estrone s.c.
** = transformation: none (0)–maximal (4)
† = active metabolite of desogestrel
1) = total dose

Investigations on androgenic activity

An important aspect of the endocrinological profile of progestogens of the 19-nortestosterone series is their androgenic activity. This property was investigated in castrated male rats (Hershberger test) and in the genitals of female rat fetuses (investigations on sexual differentiation).

Figure 6 shows a comparison of the effects of gestodene, levonorgestrel and 3-keto-desogestrel on the accessory sex glands (seminal vesicle weights). It is evident that the androgenic activity of all these substances is very slight compared to that of testosterone propionate. Effects begin to appear only at dosages three to ten times higher than those at which we would expect to observe progestogenic effects. It is surprising to find that, despite its distinctly more powerful progestogenic activity, gestodene does not possess correspondingly more potent androgenicity than levonorgestrel.

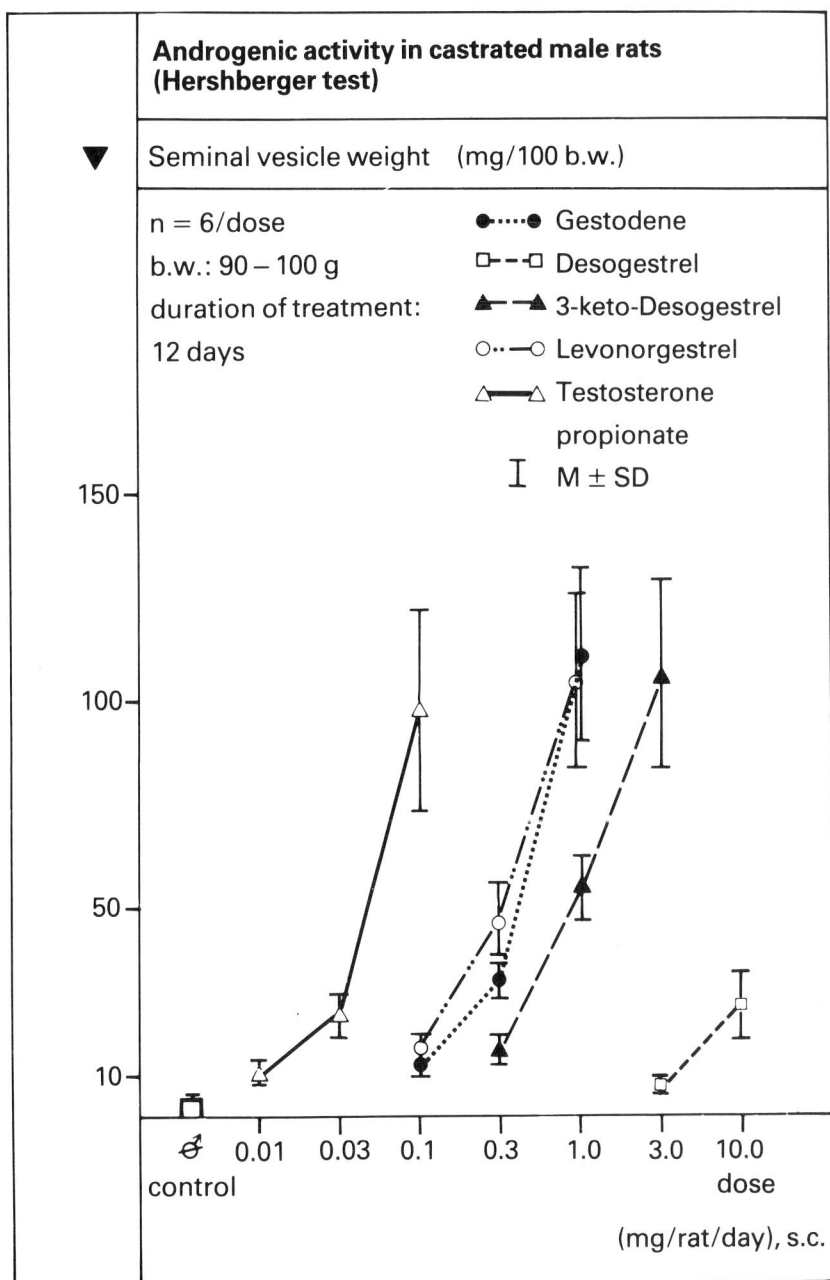

Figure 6   Changes of seminal vesicle weight in castrated male rats under treatment with various progestogens compared to testosterone propionate in the Hershberger test (modified after Ref. 17)

Now to the influence of gestodene on sexual differentiation in female rat fetuses. This test gives an indication of the transplacental effects of hormones, but is also highly specific for androgens in general.

Figure 7 sets out the basic concepts of the test. In the absence of

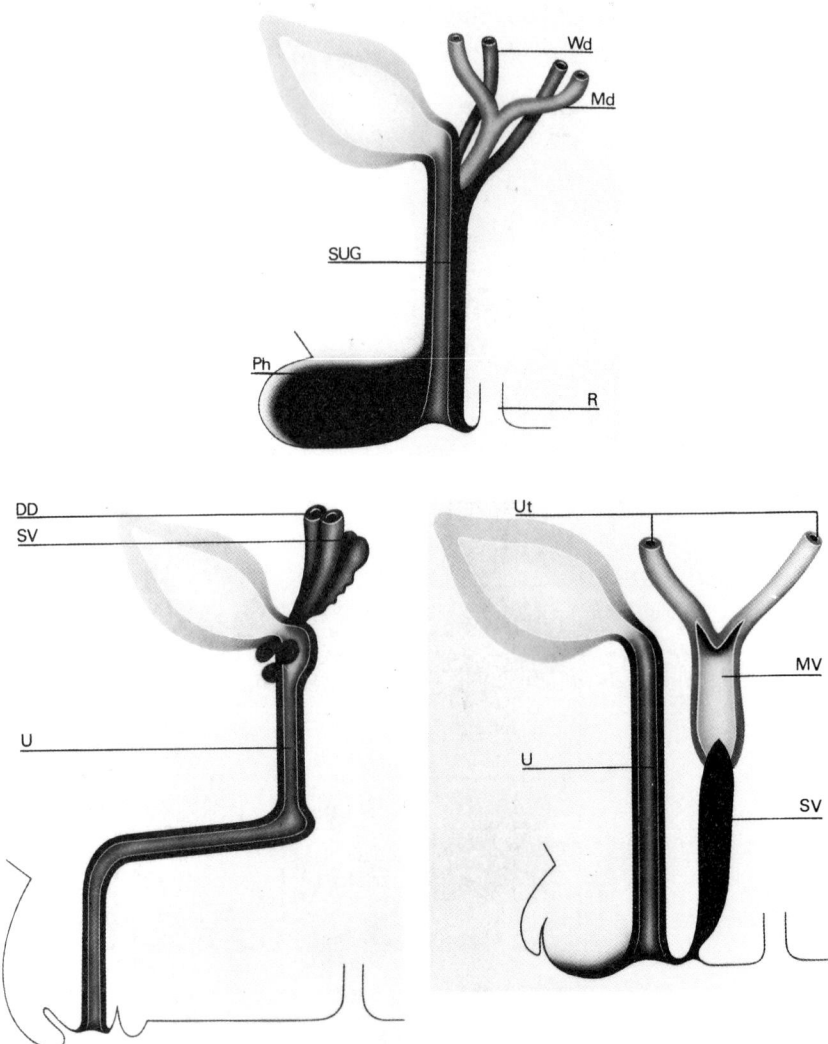

Figure 7   Bisexual stage of development of external genital organs in rats

MV	= Müllerian vagina	Ph	= Phallus + urogenital plate
SV	= Sinus vagina	Ut	= Uterus
Wd	= Wolffian ducts	U	= Urethra
Md	= Müllerian ducts	DD	= Ductus deferens
SUG	= Sinus urogenitalis	R	= Rectum

androgens the development of the undifferentiated external sex organs follows the female pattern. The sinus urogenitalis (SUG) divides into a ventral urethra and a dorsal vagina. This growth pattern is inhibited by androgens. The other morphological sex differences need not be gone into here. They are also regulated by androgens but react less sensitively than vaginal development[9-11].

Figure 8 is a comparison of levonorgestrel and gestodene. It shows

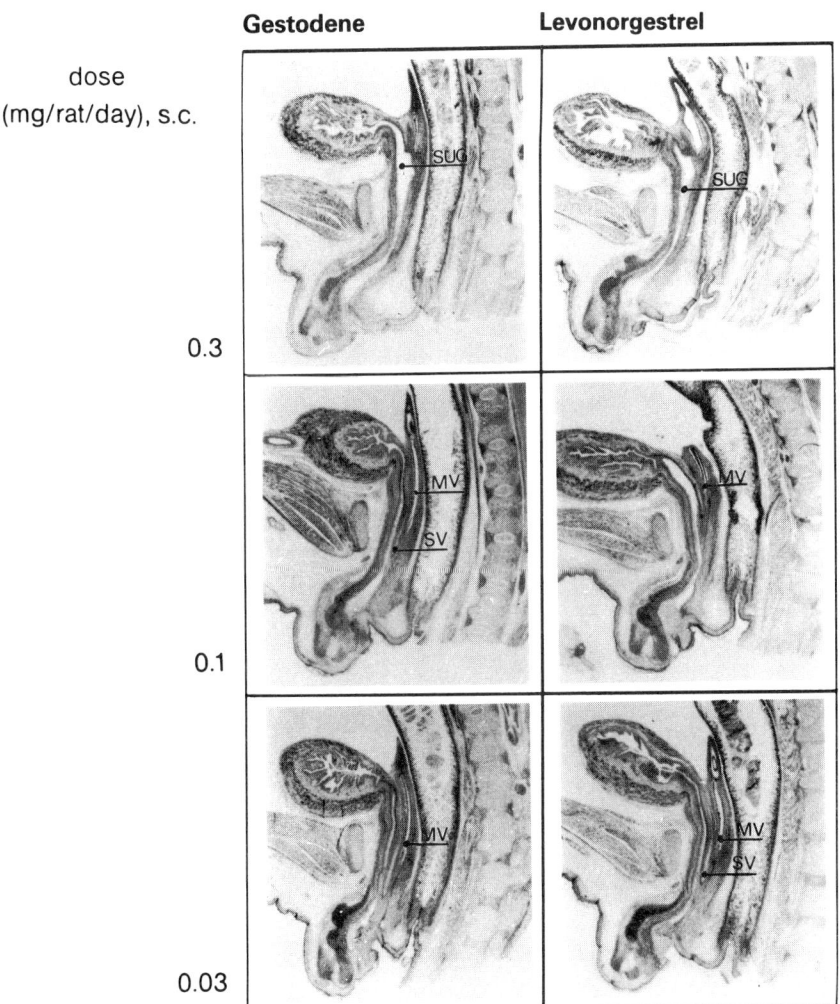

Figure 8   Sagittal section of external genital organs of day 22 female fetuses. Note: Inhibition of sinus urogenitalis (SUG) – cleavage at 0.3 mg dose level. Smaller degree of transformation at 0.1 mg dose level; gestodene < levonorgestrel. Normal female development at the 0.03 mg/animal/day s.c. dose level for both compounds

that doses of 0.03 mg/dam/day s.c. of these two substances lead to completely normal development of the vagina with a section which divides off from the Müllerian duct and a caudal section leading off from the SUG. A ten-fold increase in the dose, to 0.3 mg/dam/day s.c., of both substances severely inhibited the development of a vagina. At 0.1 mg/dam/day differences appear which indicate a somewhat lower absolute androgenicity of gestodene as compared to levonorgestrel in this trial design.

At this dose (0.1 mg/day s.c.) there is predominantly normal development of the vagina under gestodene, whereas the majority of the fetuses under levonorgestrel exhibit partial inhibition.

Relationship between progestogenic and androgenic activity in animal studies

Figure 9 illustrates the doses in gravid rats at which progestogenic (= pregnancy-maintaining) and minimal masculinizing (= androgenic) effects become evident in female fetuses.

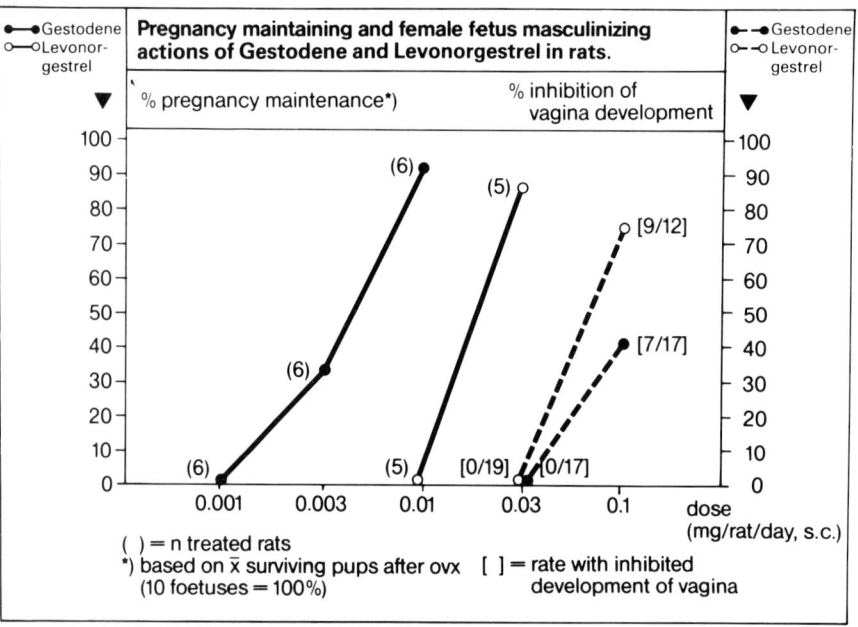

Figure 9   Progestogenic, i.e., pregnancy maintaining, and androgenic, i.e., masculinizing, activities of gestodene compared to those of levonorgestrel

In the pregnancy maintenance test even doses of gestodene and levonorgestrel which elicit their full progestogenic potency do not influence the sexual development of female fetuses. It is, however, also readily apparent that the degree of separation between progestogenic and androgenic activity is much greater in respect of gestodene than in the case of levonorgestrel. In other words, these findings confirm that in relation to its main activity gestodene is less androgenic than levonorgestrel.

Anti-estrogenic effects

An important aspect of the activity profile of a progestogen is, as already stated, its ability to suppress estrogenic activity. Depending on which target organ or function is concerned, it is possible that various other hormone characteristics apart from the progestogenic activity itself, i.e., its androgenic properties, play an important part.

Figure 10 shows an example of an anti-estrogenic model – the sialic acid test in the mouse – in which both progestogenic and androgenic

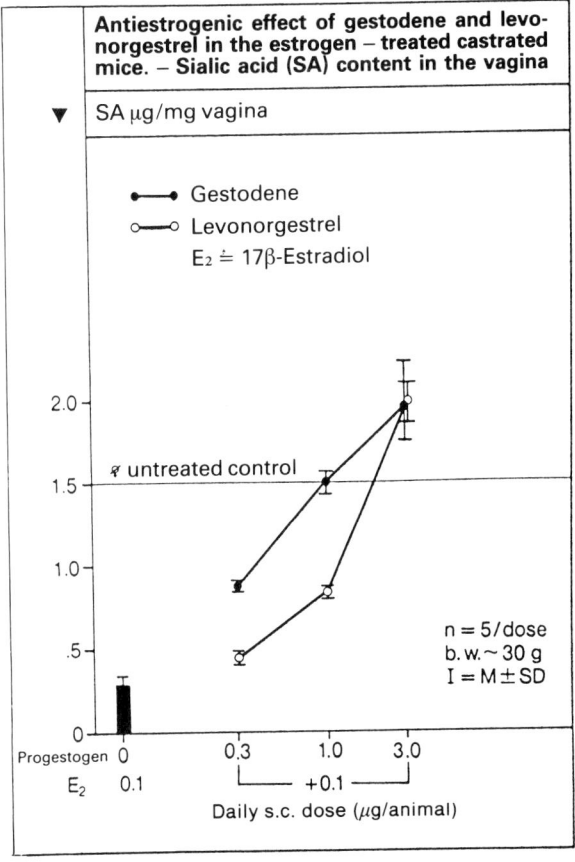

Figure 10   *Anti-estrogenic activity of gestodene and levonorgestrel at the vagina of ovariectomized adult mice (modified after Ref. 17)*

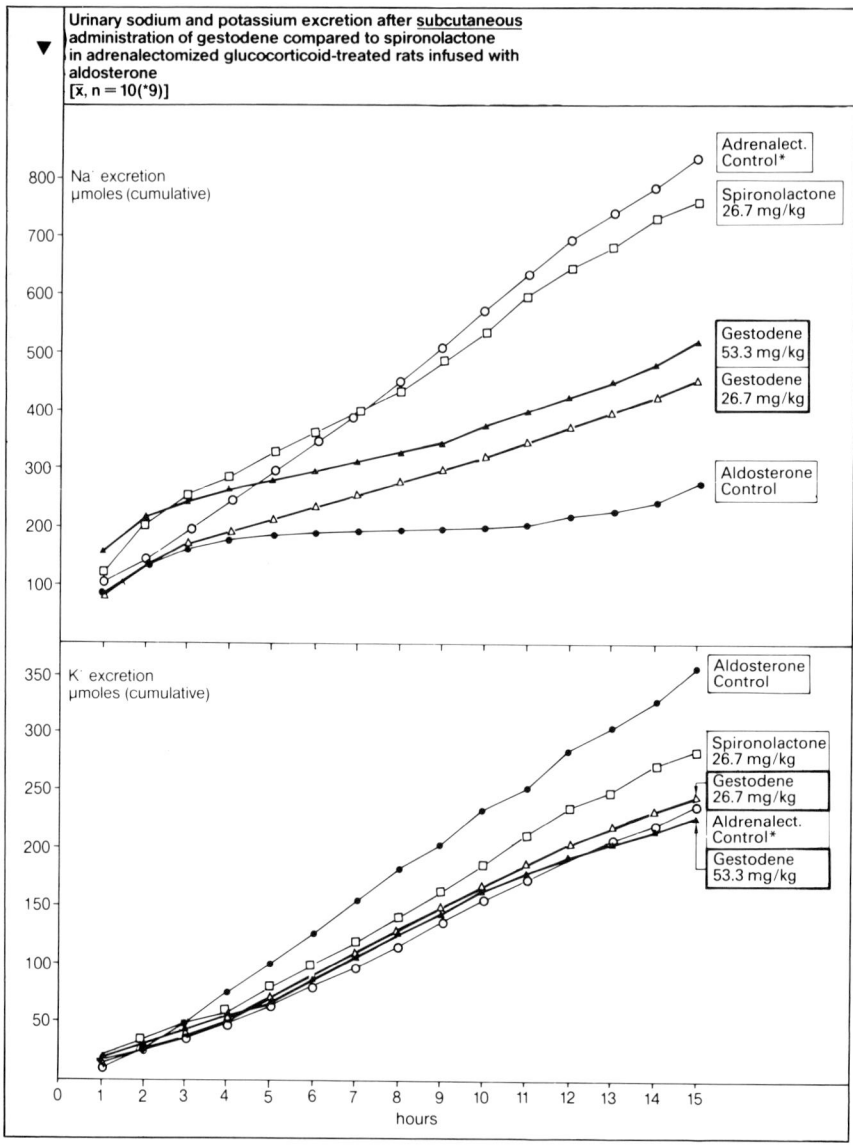

▼ Urinary sodium and potassium excretion after <u>subcutaneous</u>
administration of gestodene compared to spironolactone
in adrenalectomized glucocorticoid-treated rats infused with
aldosterone
[x̄, n = 10(*9)]

Figure 11   Urinary sodium and potassium excretion after subcutaneous administration of gestodene compared to spironolactone in adrenalectomized glucocorticoid-treated rats infused with aldosterone (modified after Ref. 12)

effects can play a part. Estrogens lower the level of sialic acid in the vagina of spayed animals. Progestogens negate this effect in a dose-dependent manner. This experiment showed that gestodene's capacity to suppress estrogenic effects tends to be higher than that of levonorgestrel in absolute terms. Because of the more potent progestogenic activity of gestodene this difference should be regarded as relative.

Other effects of gestodene

In conclusion, attention should be drawn to a property of gestodene which distinguishes it from all previous progestogens. Mention was made at the start of this article of the fact that gestodene has a surprisingly high affinity for the aldosterone receptor (Table 1). This affinity corresponds to weak anti-aldosterone activity in adrenalectomized rats[12] in which aldosterone partially blocks the elimination of sodium with the urine (Figure 11).

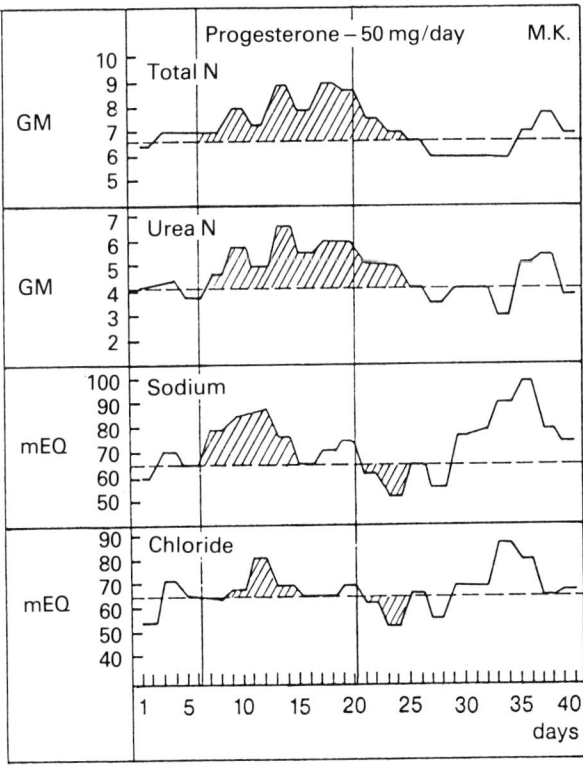

Figure 12   Effect of progesterone administered intramuscularly on the excretion of several urinary constituents in a young woman (modified after Ref. 13)

In this respect gestodene can be compared with progesterone which, in physiological doses, has a natriuretic effect *in man* (Figure 12)[13-16].

CONCLUSIONS

(1) Gestodene is probably the most powerful progestogen known in humans and animals. Its biochemical profile in respect of binding sites for steroid hormones is very similar to that of progesterone. The same applies to its hormonal properties.

(2) In absolute terms and in relation to its main, i.e., its progestogenic, activity it possesses very little androgenic potency.

(3) The data presented indicate that gestodene possesses anti-estrogenic activity corresponding to its high progestogenic efficacy.

(4) Gestodene has virtually no estrogenic or glucocorticoid activity.

(5) Gestodene's aldosterone-antagonistic activity is a new property. It is doubtful whether this can have any clinical significance, but it does help to underline the similarity between the action of the gestodene molecule and progesterone.

REFERENCES

1. Gaspard, U. J. (1983). In V. R. Mahesh and R. B. Greenblatt (eds) *Role of Anti-androgens in the Treatment of Acne*, pp 369–94. John Wright – PSG Inc.

2. Hammerstein, J., Lachnit-Fixson, U., Neumann, F. and Plewig, G. (eds) (1980). *Androgenization in Women – Acne, Seborrhoea, Androgenetic Alopecia and Hirsutism*. Excerpta Medica, Amsterdam, Oxford and Princeton.

3. Lachnit-Fixson, U. (1982). Development and clinical evaluation of triphasic oral contraception. In M. Elstein (ed.) *Update on Triphasic Oral Contraception*, pp 37–53. Excerpta Medica.

4. Hofmeister, H., Wiechert, R., Annen, K., Laurent, H. and Steinbeck, H. (1975). DE 25.46.062/10 Okt. (*Chem. Abstracts 87*, 168265k/1977).

5. Hofmeister, H., Annen, K., Laurent, H., Petzoldt, K. and Wiechert, R. Synthesen von 17d-ethinyl-17β-hydroxy-18-methyl-4, 15-estradien-3-on. (In preparation).

6. Gaspard, U. J. (1985). Serum lipid and lipid protein changes induced by new oral contraceptives containing ethinyl-estradiol plus levonorgestrel or desogestrel. *Contraception, 31*, 395–409.

7. Pollow, K. and co-workers (1983/84). Unpublished data.

8. Beier, S., Düsterberg, B., El Etreby, M. F., Elger, W., Neumann, F. and Nishino, Y. (1983). Toxicology of hormonal fertility-regulating agents. In G. Benagiano and E. Diczfalusy (eds) *Endocrine Mechanisms in Fertility-Regulation*, pp 261–346. Raven Press, New York.

9. Jost, A. (1946). III. Rôle des gonades foetales dans la différenciation sexuelle somatique. *Arch. Anat. Microsc. Morphol. Exp., 36*, 271.

10. Hamada, H., Neumann, F. und Junkmann, K. (1963). Intrauterine antimaskuline Beeinflussung von Rattenfeten durch ein stark Gestagen-wirksames Steroid. *Acta Endocrinol. (Kopenhagen), 44*, 350.

11. Elger, W. (1966). Die Rolle der fetalen Androgene in der Sexualdifferenzierung des Kaninchens und ihre Abgrenzung gegen andere hormonale und somatische Faktoren durch Anwendung eines starken Antiandrogens. *Arch. Anat. Microsc. Morphol. Ex.*, **55**, 657.

12. Losert, W., Casals-Stenzel, J. and Buse, M. (1985). Progestogens with anti-mineralocorticoid activity. *Drug Res.*, **35**, 459–471.

13. Landau, R. L., Bergenstal, D. M., Lugibihl, K. and Kascht, M. E. (1955). The metabolic effects of progesterone in man. *J. Clin. Endocrinol. Metab.*, **15**, 1194.

14. Landau, R. L. and Lugibihl, K. (1958). Inhibition of the sodium-retaining influence of aldosterone by progesterone. *J. Clin. Endocrinol. Metab.*, **18**, 1237.

15. Landau, R. L. and Lugibihl, K. (1961). The catabolic and natriuretic effects of progesterone in man. *Rec. Prog. Horm. Res.*, **17**, 249.

16. Wambach, G. and Higgins, J. R. (1979). Antimineralocorticoid action of progesterone. In M. K. Agarwal (ed.) *Antihormones*, p. 167. Elsevier North-Holland, Biomedical Press, Amsterdam.

17. Nishino, Y. (1985). Unpublished data of Schering AG, Berlin/Bergkamen.

2

Pharmacokinetics and biotransformation of gestodene in man

B. Düsterberg, J.-W. Tack, W. Krause and M. Hümpel

The special pharmacokinetic properties of gestodene as observed in women can be reported based in the main on the results of three studies.

The design of the first study is represented in Table 1. Gestodene was administered both intravenously and orally, as a single dosage of

Table 1   Design of pharmacokinetic study 1 with gestodene on healthy female volunteers

n	Dose	Route of administration	Pharmaceutic preparation	Regimen	Aim of the study, pharmacokinetic parameters to be investigated
6	75 μg gestodene	Intravenous	Solution	Single administration	Absorption, bioavailability, time-course of the gestodene level in plasma
6	75 μg gestodene + 30 μg ethinyl estradiol	Oral	Coated tablet	Single administration	

75 μg each. The doses were administered one after the other after an interval of 6 days in the same subjects. Intravenous injection would appear unusual but is a precondition in particular for determining the oral bioavailability of gestodene. The goal of the investigations was to permit conclusions to be drawn on the absorption, the bioavailability and the time-course of the concentration of the active ingredient in plasma. Sensitive and specific methods of analysis for the substance to be determined are the prerequisite for determining the pharmacokinetic parameters mentioned.

Since gestodene was administered in very low doses, only two methods lent themselves for application, namely, radio-immunological determination of the active ingredient in plasma and measurement of radioactivity (Table 2) when, as was the case in the third study, the radioactively labelled drug was administered.

Table 2   Analytical methods for the determination of the concentration of gestodene in biological samples

1.   Specific radio-immunoassay for the metabolically unchanged drug in plasma
2.   Measurement of radioactivity in plasma, urine and feces following the administration of ^{14}C-gestodene (scintillation-counting)

The results of the first study can be illustrated (Figure 1) on the basis of the curve of the active ingredient concentrations after intravenous and oral administration of, in each case, a single dose of the preparation.

As expected, the maximum concentration of gestodene in plasma was determined immediately after the end of injection. Thereafter the gestodene level dropped in three phases with half-life periods of an average of 10 minutes, 1.5 and 10 hours.

After oral administration the gestodene was absorbed rapidly with a half-life value of about one hour. The maximum active ingredient levels were recorded 1–2 hours after swallowing. Thereafter, two phases were demonstrated in the rate of decline of the gestodene level, with half-life periods of approximately 1 and 12 hours. The half-life periods determined after intravenous and oral administration coincide well.

The bioavailability, by virtue of its definition, is the percentage of a dose administered orally which reaches the general circulatory system. The intravenous dose can in this connection be considered to be completely bioavailable, i.e., to an extent of 100%, and may serve as a reference for the oral form of administration.

On the basis of this comparison, which in practice was made via the areas under the active ingredient levels after the two types of administration, it was possible to demonstrate complete bioavailability for gestodene after oral administration (Figure 2).

In the second study (Table 3) the pharmacokinetic behaviour of gestodene under normal administration conditions was investigated, i.e., over a 21-day treatment period. The dosage again amounted to 75 μg, which was administered in combination with 30 μg ethinyl estradiol daily at the same time of day to 6 young test women. The objective of the second study was above all to shed light on the

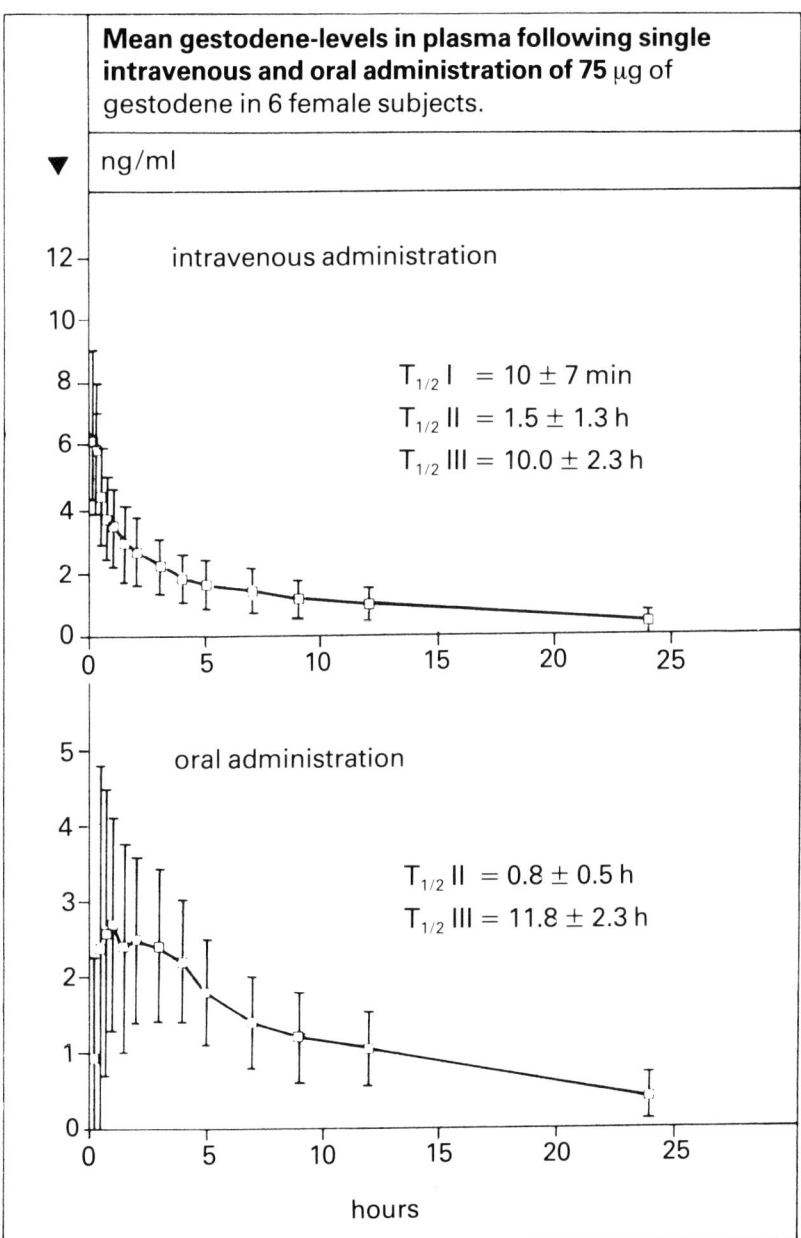

Figure 1   *Mean gestodene levels in plasma following single intravenous and oral administration of 75 μg of gestodene in 6 female subjects.*

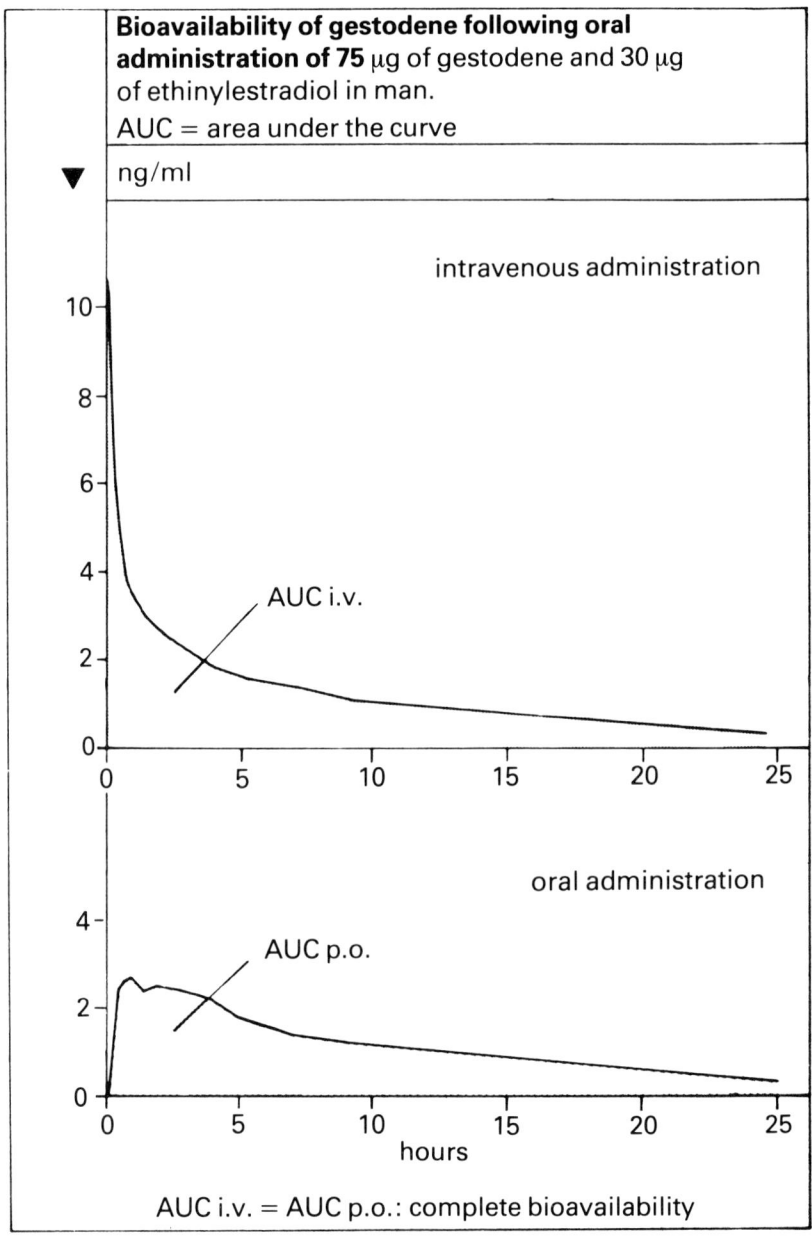

Figure 2   Bioavailability of gestodene following oral administration of 75 µg of ges-todene and 30 µg of ethinyl estradiol in man. AUC = area under the curve

Table 3   Design of pharmacokinetic study 2 with gestodene on healthy female volunteers

n	Dose	Route of administration	Pharmaceutic preparation	Dose regimen	Aim of the study, pharmacokinetic parameters to be investigated
6	75 μg gestodene + 30 μg ethinyl estradiol	Oral	Coated tablet	Daily administration for 21 days	Time course of the drug level in plasma, accumulation

question as to whether under the normal treatment scheme for an oral contraceptive changes in the pharmacokinetics of gestodene occur and whether cumulative processes might become evident due to a clear increase in the active ingredient level in the plasma.

As will be seen from the graphic representation (Figure 3) of results in a test subject, the gestodene level, measured in each case 24 hours after administration, increased under daily oral administration of the test preparation and reached maximum values within a period ranging from the 14th to the 19th day. In the course of the last days of administration, no further rise in the gestodene level was established.

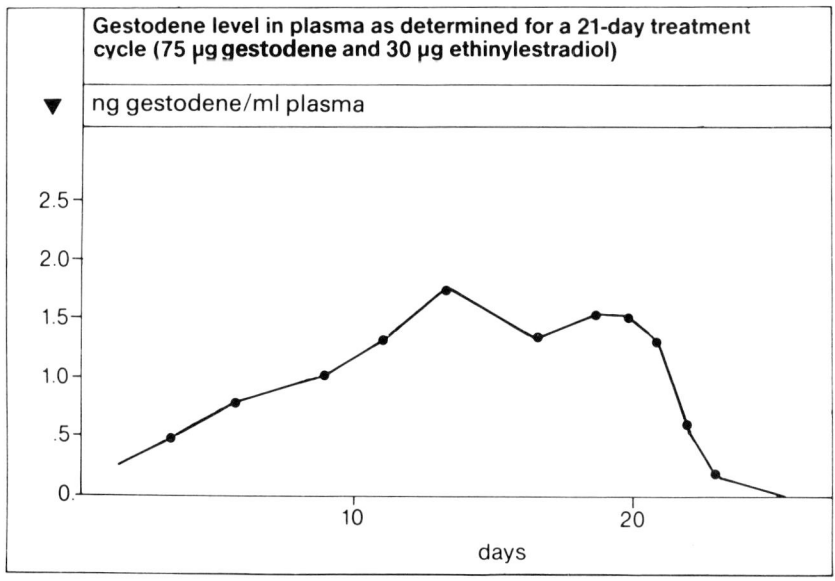

Figure 3   Gestodene level in plasma as determined for a 21-day treatment cycle (75 μg gestodene and 30 μg ethinyl estradiol) in one test subject

After administration of the last dose, i.e., after the 21st day, a declining gestodene level was observed analogous to the first study.

The half-life periods (Figure 4) calculated after administration of the 21st dose were markedly longer than after a single dose of gestodene

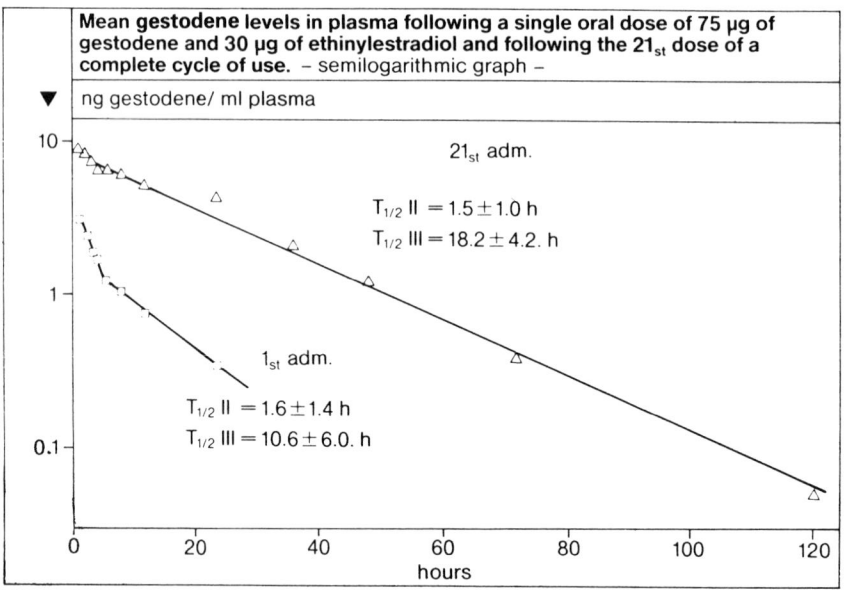

Figure 4   *Mean gestodene levels in plasma following a single oral dose of 75 μg of gestodene and 30 μg of ethinyl estradiol and following the 21st dose of a complete cycle of use*

and exhibited average values of 1.5 to 18.2 hours. In the graphic representation the concentrations are plotted semilogarithmically in order to make clear the various phases of elimination with the related half-life periods.

As a reason for the observed increase in the gestodene level in the course of a cycle of administration and of the prolonged terminal half-life periods after the last dose, cumulative processes could be assumed which, however, would demand as a prerequisite a markedly longer terminal half-life period than that observed. It thus appeared more appropriate to assume that the binding capacity of the plasma proteins altered during the course of administration.

In the course of a preliminary cycle and the treatment cycle, the concentration of SHBG, i.e., the sex-hormone-binding globulin, was determined in the plasma (Figure 5). As will be seen from the illustration, which is based on the example of a test woman, the SHBG level increased quite clearly. As a result of this the gestodene level

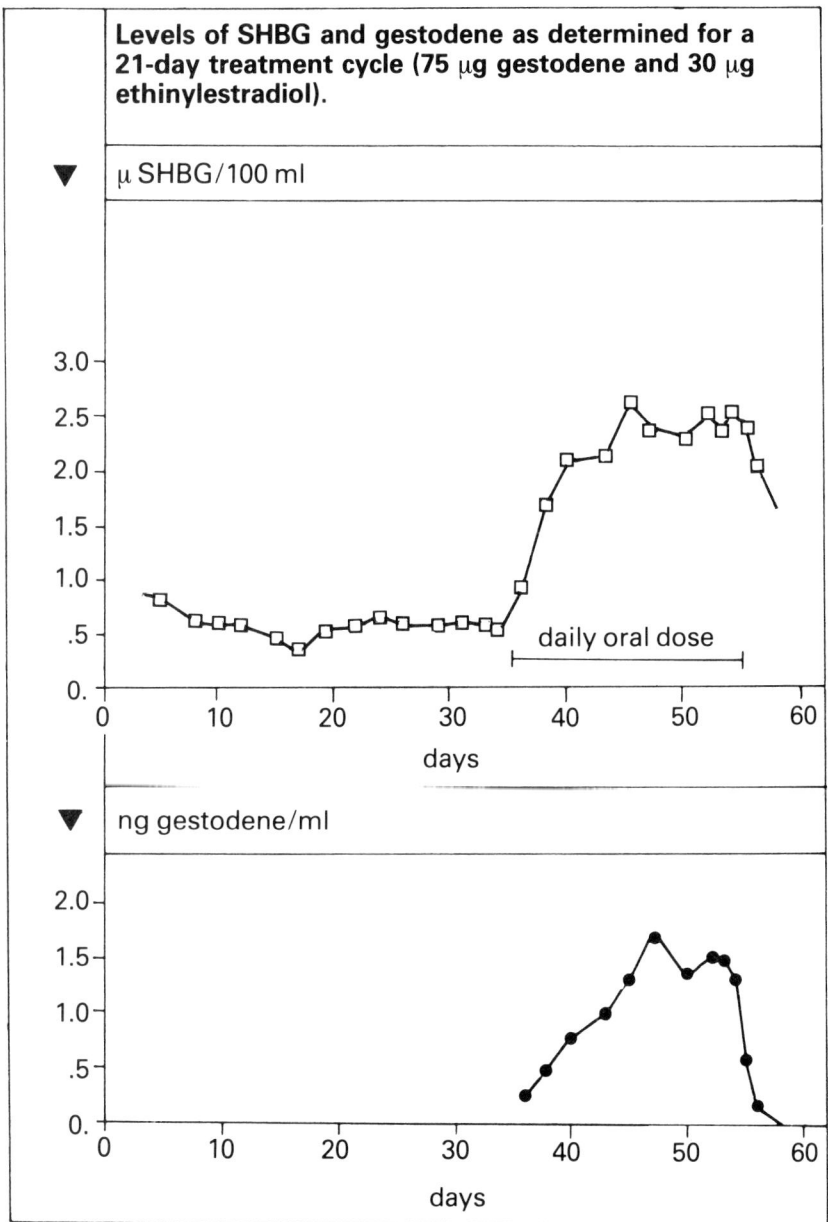

Figure 5   Plasma levels of SHBG and gestodene as determined for a 21-day treatment cycle (75 µg gestodene and 30 µg ethinyl estradiol) in one test subject

Table 4   Design of pharmacokinetic study 3 with gestodene on healthy female volunteers

n	Dose	Route of administration	Pharmaceutic preparation	Dose regimen	Aim of the study, pharmacokinetic parameters to be investigated
3	500 μg ^{14}C- gestodene	oral	Capsule	Single administration	Metabolic pattern in urine, identification of metabolites, excretion of the drug

certainly rose likewise. The cause of the change in the protein concentration, on the other hand, is the ethinyl estradiol contained in the preparation under test, for which this inducing effect has long been known.

The third series of studies (Table 4) was intended to shed light on biotransformation and elimination of this progestogen. Three women were given a single oral dose of 500 μg of ^{14}C-labelled gestodene.

The spectrum of the radioactively labelled metabolites in urine was determined with the aid of high pressure chromatography (Figure 6).

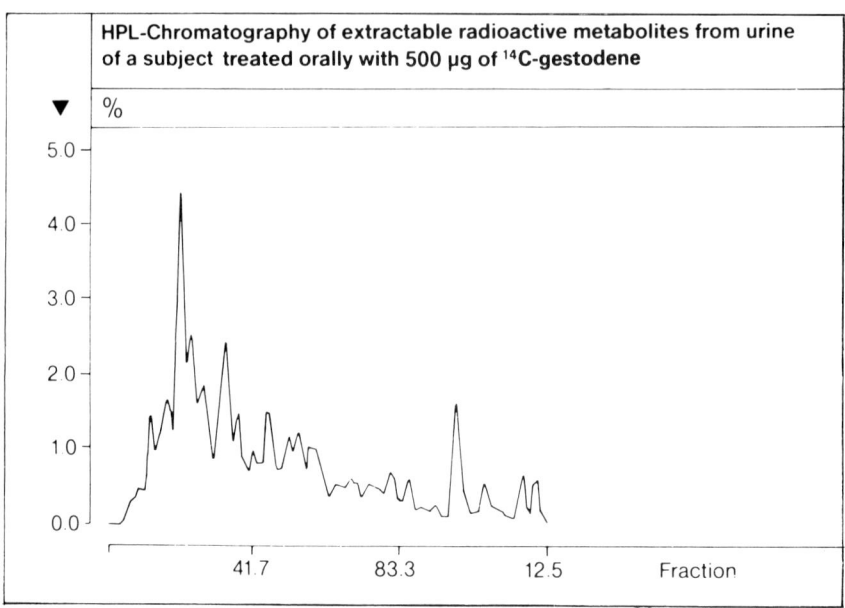

Figure 6   *HPL-chromatography of extractable radioactive metabolites from urine of a subject treated orally with 500 μg of ^{14}C-gestodene*

Chemical structure of metabolites formed from gestodene in man

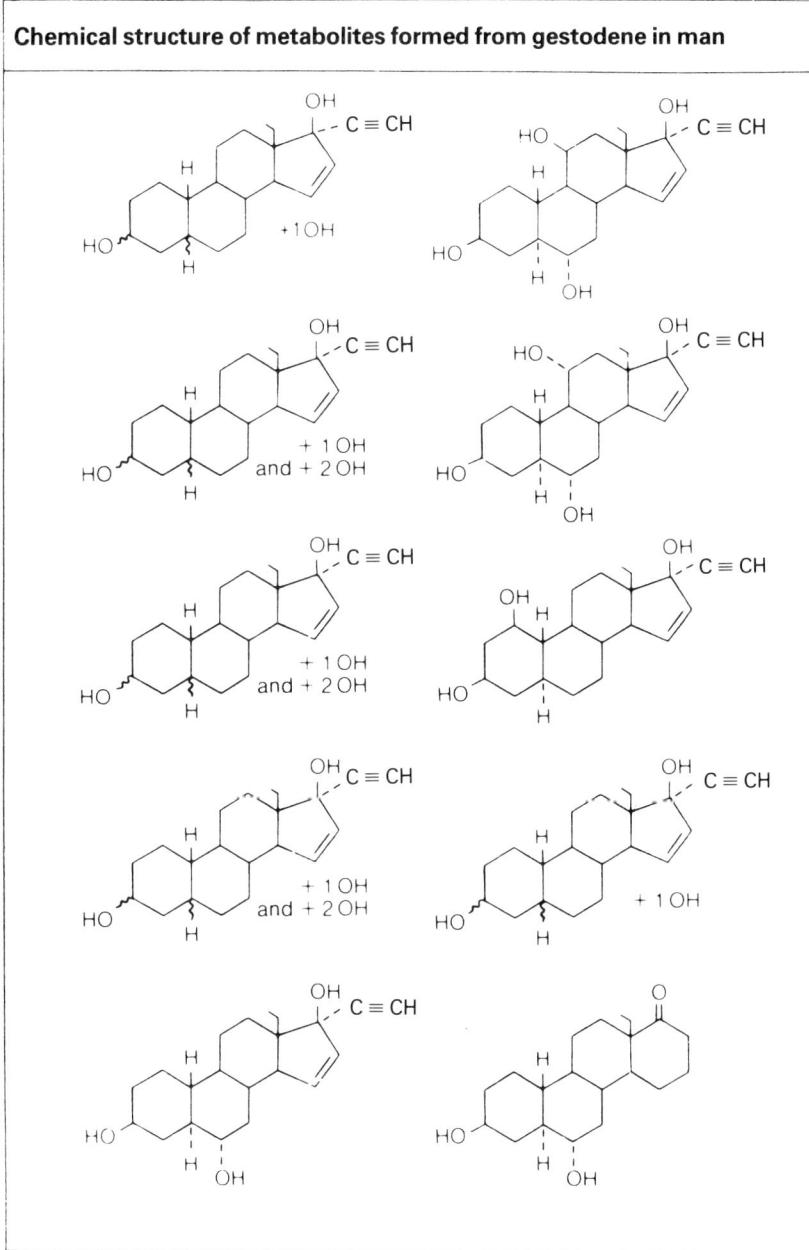

Figure 7   Chemical structure of metabolites formed from gestodene in man. (Some of the compounds contain one or two hydroxy-groups in addition; however, the precise structure remains unclear)

This shows the radioactivity peaks contained in the individual fractions, which in each case contain at least one gestodene metabolite. Similar to many other steroids, gestodene is converted into a large number of metabolites *in vivo*.

It was possible to isolate some of the metabolites from urine by various biochemical analytical methods and to identify them (Figure 7). All metabolites identified are steroids with higher polarity than gestodene and are produced by oxidation and reduction processes. The reduction process occurred on the 3-keto group as well as the Δ^4-double bond. Hydroxylation took place at various points of the molecule. In the case of one metabolite, the 17α-ethinyl group was changed, which was reflected in the expansion of the D pentagonal ring to a D hexagonal ring. In the case of all the structures elucidated, apart from the last mentioned exception, both the Δ^{15}-double bond as well as the C17-ethinyl group remained intact.

Gestodene is practically not excreted at all in an unchanged form. In the form of metabolites the ^{14}C-gestodene was eliminated via the

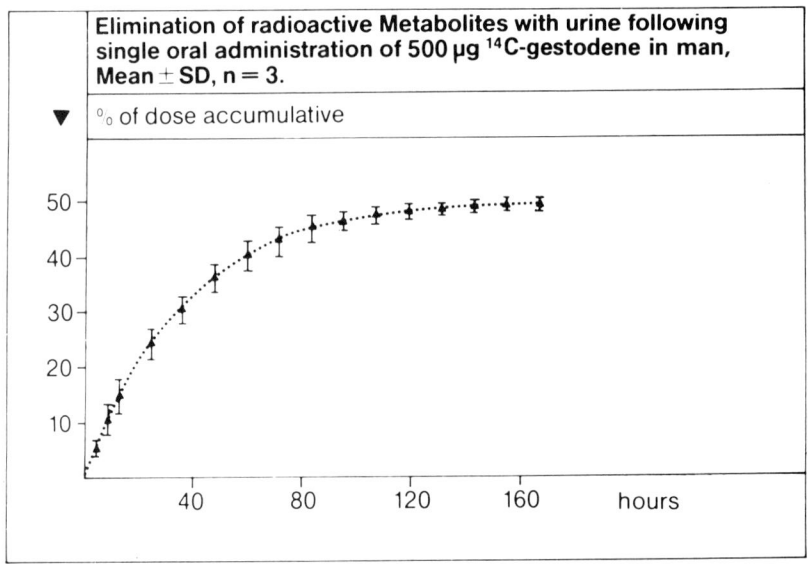

Figure 8   Elimination of radioactive metabolites with urine following single oral administration of 500 μg ^{14}C-gestodene in man. Mean ± SD, n = 3

kidneys to an extent of 50% of the dose given. Excretion was in a phase with a half-life period of about one day (Figure 8). Seven days after administration of a single dose of the progestogen, elimination by urine and faeces was complete.

3

Inhibition of ovulation with gestodene

J. Spona and J. Huber

SUMMARY

Gestodene was tested to its effect as a progestogen. In addition, the ovulation inhibition dosage was determined for this new generation progestogen. Gestodene showed no affinity for the estrogen receptor. The relative binding affinity (RBA) for the progestogen receptor of the rat uterus was greater in the case of gestodene than for levonorgestrel and desogestrel. For gestodene a slightly larger affinity towards the androgen receptor was established than for desogestrel and levonorgestrel, whereas the biological activity, which was examined on the basis of the β-glucuronidase activity, was similar to that of desogestrel and levonorgestrel. Experiments on the modulation of gonadotropin release following stimulation by LH-RH showed that gestodene exhibited a greater progestogenic effect than levonorgestrel. 40 μg was found as a value for the ovulation inhibition dosage for gestodene. This limiting dosage is less than that of levonorgestrel. The results of these investigations show that gestodene, in comparison to progestogens used hitherto in oral contraceptives, is biologically more active and thus permits reduction in the dosage. Moreover, gestodene shows a low androgenic effect similar to that of desogestrel.

INTRODUCTION

Developments in the field of new oral contraceptives have in recent years mainly been characterized by devising new dosaging schemes. This has led to the concept of the triphasic pill[1]. Development of a new progestogen[2] likewise led to development of a low-dose combination preparation. The aim of this research work is to develop contraceptives which exhibit a minimum dose of estrogen and progestogen. By this means side-effects on the parameters of the hemostatic system and metabolic functions would be kept as low as possible. The World Health

Organization (WHO) issued such a recommendation as early as 1978 with this objective in mind.

In the present investigation we report on results which led to the development of gestodene. The present report sums up preclinical studies.

MATERIAL AND METHODS

Determination of the relative binding affinity (RBA)

The RBA was examined for the estrogen receptor (ER), the pro-gesterone receptor (PgR) and the androgen receptor (AR). The method of determining the RBA of the three above-mentioned receptors has been described by us in detail[4]. For examination of ER and PgR, cytosol preparations from rat uteri were resorted to. Determination of AR was carried out with the aid of cytosol preparations from mouse kidneys. ^{3}H-labelled R 5020, estradiol and R 1881 were employed as ligands.

Determination of β-glucuronidase activity

Results of examinations on the stimulation of β-glucuronidase activity were resorted to as parameters for determination of the androgenicity of progestogens[5]. The method has already been described by us in detail[4].

Determination of the modulation of gonadotropin release induced by LH-RH

Progestogen modulation of the LH and FSH release induced by LH-RH was examined *in vivo* on the basis of a rat test and *in vitro* in a hypophyseal cell culture system. These two model systems serve for determining the biological potency of gestodene with respect to its hypophyseal effect. For this purpose ovariectomized rats were injected subcutaneously for 7 days with various doses of progestogens and 24 hours after the last dose of progestogen had been administered they were injected i.p. with 200 ng of LH-RH. After 30 minutes a blood sample was taken by cardiopuncture and rLH and rFSH were deter-mined by radio-immunoassay.

The *in vitro* effect was tested in a primary cell culture in hypophyses. The incubation took place with increasing concentrations of LH-RH in the presence or absence of the relevant progestogen. The rLH and rFSH concentrations in the medium were examined radio-immunologically. This work has already been reported in detail[6].

Determination of the ovulation inhibition dosage

The ovulation inhibition dosage for gestodene was determined in the case of 23 women, aged from 20 to 28, with normal cycles. After one control cycle the test subjects were given a daily oral dose of 10, 20, 30 and 40 μg of gestodene from day 5 to day 25 of the cycle. During the control cycle and the cycle under investigation, LH, FSH, 17β-estradiol and progesterone were examined by radio-immunoassay. Likewise, the cervical score and the karyopyknotic index were recorded.

Examination of ovulation inhibition with a combination preparation

A total of 10 test subjects with normal cycles were treated after one control cycle with a daily oral dose of 75 μg of gestodene + 30 μg of ethinyl estradiol from the 5th to the 25th day of the cycle. LH, FSH, 17β-estradiol, progesterone and prolactin were measured by radio-immunoassay.

RESULTS

Receptor interactions

Investigations into the relative binding affinity (RBA) showed that gestodene exhibits no affinity to the estrogen receptor.

However, a greater RBA was found for gestodene for the interaction with the progestogen receptor of the rat uterus than for levonorgestrel and desogestrel. These results (Table 1) mean that gestodene exhibits

Table 1 Relative binding affinity (RBA) for the interaction of levonorgestrel, desogestrel and gestodene with the progesterone receptor of the rat uterus

	RBA (R5020)
Levonorgestrel	0.1276 ± 0.0289
Desogestrel	1.2996 ± 0.2544
Gestodene	2.3410 ± 0.3989

a greater affinity towards the progestogen receptor than the two other progestogens examined. On the other hand, in the mouse kidney model system, a greater affinity towards the androgen receptor was established than for desogestrel and levonorgestrel (Figure 1).

Biological activity of gestodene

The biological activity of levonorgestrel, desogestrel and gestodene was compared in the mouse kidney model system employed. Stimulation of the β-glucuronidase activity is a measure of the androgenicity of a progestogen. The results (Figure 2) show that gestodene in the higher dosage range exhibits an androgenicity level similar to that of desogestrel.

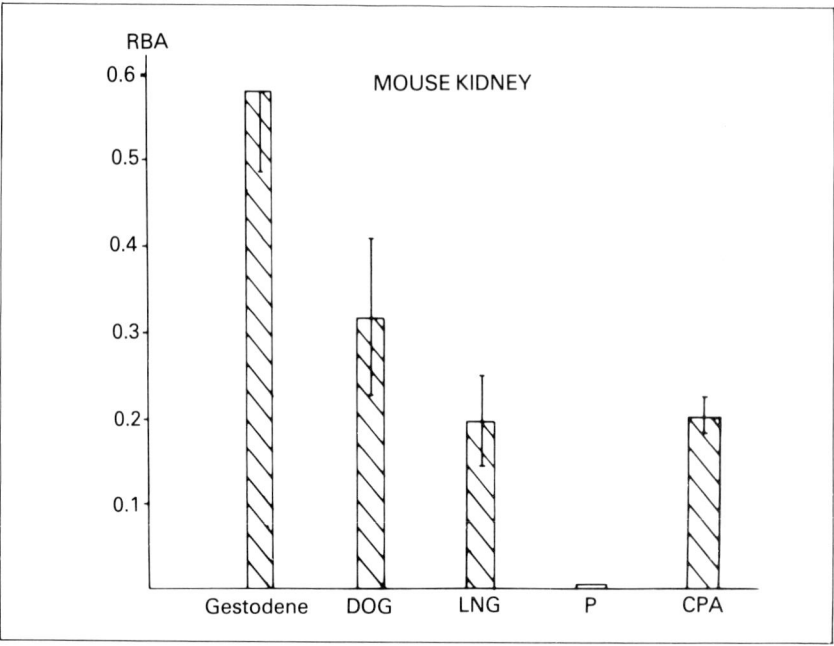

Figure 1   Relative binding affinity for the androgen receptor in mouse kidney cytosol

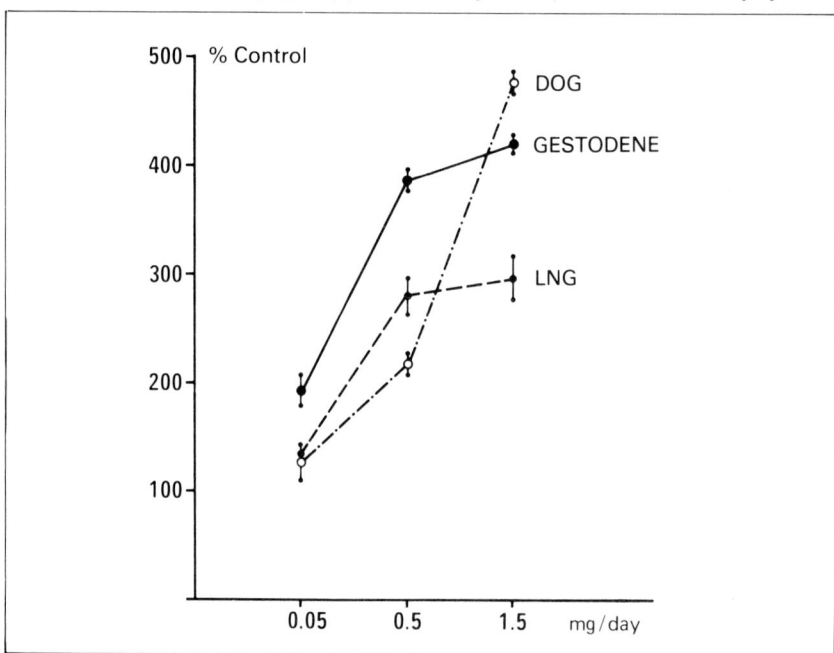

Figure 2   Glucuronidase activity after s.c. application of levonorgestrel (LNG), gestodene and desogestrel (DOG)

Modulation of LH-RH effect

Treatment of adult ovariectomized rats with gestodene did not lead to a change in the basal LH serum levels (Figure 3). On the other hand, an increase in the LH serum level following stimulation by LH-RH was observed. It was shown that a dose of 100 μg of gestodene brought about LH release after stimulation with LH-RH, which was similar to that which could be observed under 300 μg of levonorgestrel. Likewise, a dose of levonorgestrel three times as large in comparison to gestodene was necessary to suppress the FSH release by stimulation with LH-RH. The conclusion can thus be drawn that gestodene possesses biological activity three times higher than that of levonorgestrel.

Experiments with a primary cell culture comprised of rat pituitaries showed that the progestogens examined in this system brought about inhibition of gonadotropin release following stimulation by LH-RH (Figure 4). Levonorgestrel suppressed the LH release to 40% and the FSH secretion to 50% at ED_{50} of LH-RH. In a similar manner gestodene at ED_{50} of LH-RH suppressed LH and FSH release to a level of 50–70% (Figure 4). These experiments likewise point towards higher biological activity in the case of gestodene in comparison with levonorgestrel.

Ovulation inhibition dosage

The results with regard to determining the ovulation inhibition dosage are summed up in Table 2. At a dosage of 40 μg inhibition of ovulation

Table 2 Determination of the ovulation inhibition dosage of gestodene

Dose (μg)	Number of subjects	Inhibition of ovulation	With follicular maturation	Luteal insuffi- ciency	Normal cycle
10	2	–	–	2	–
20	2	–	–	1	1
30	12	11	8	–	1
40	7	6	4	1	–

was found in 6 out of 7 of the women studied. In the case of one test subject, although ovulation occurred luteal insufficiency was present. Four out of 6 anovulatory cycles showed some evidence of follicle stimulation. Thus 40 μg gestodene is considered to be the limiting dosage for ovulation inhibition. Examination of the peripheral cycle parameters showed that in all cycles – i.e., even with the 10 μg dosage – inhibition of the cervical score and the karyopyknotic index was observed.

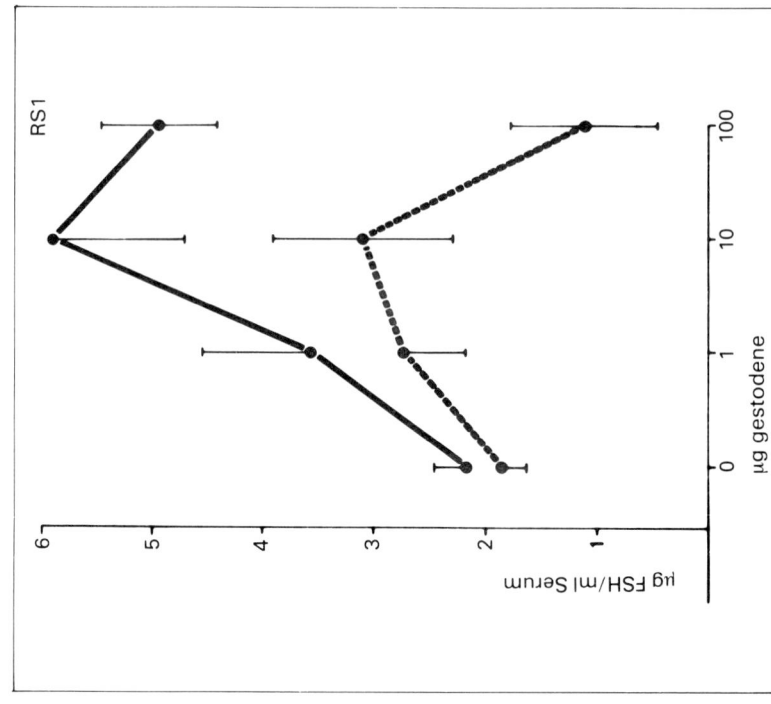

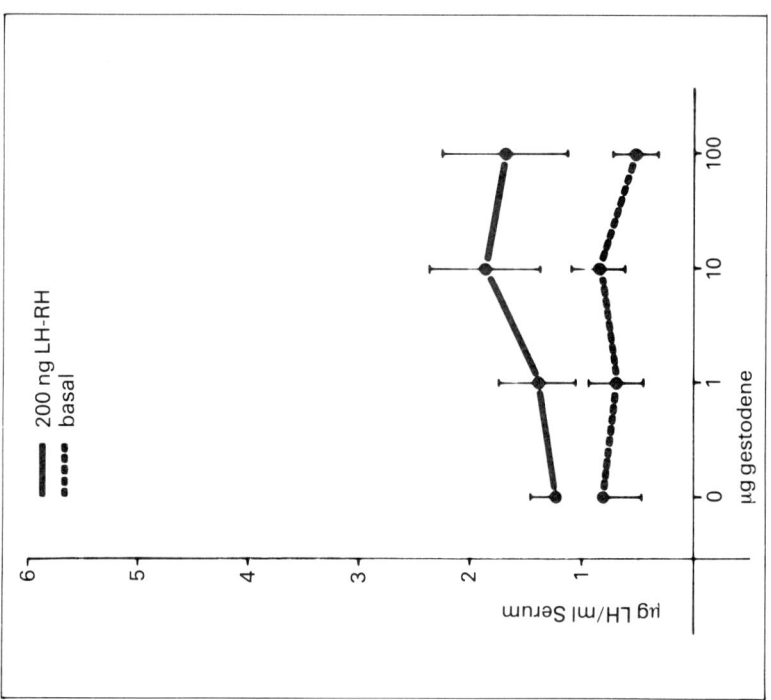

Figure 3   Modulation of LH and FSH serum levels following stimulation by LH-RH in the case of ovariectomized rats

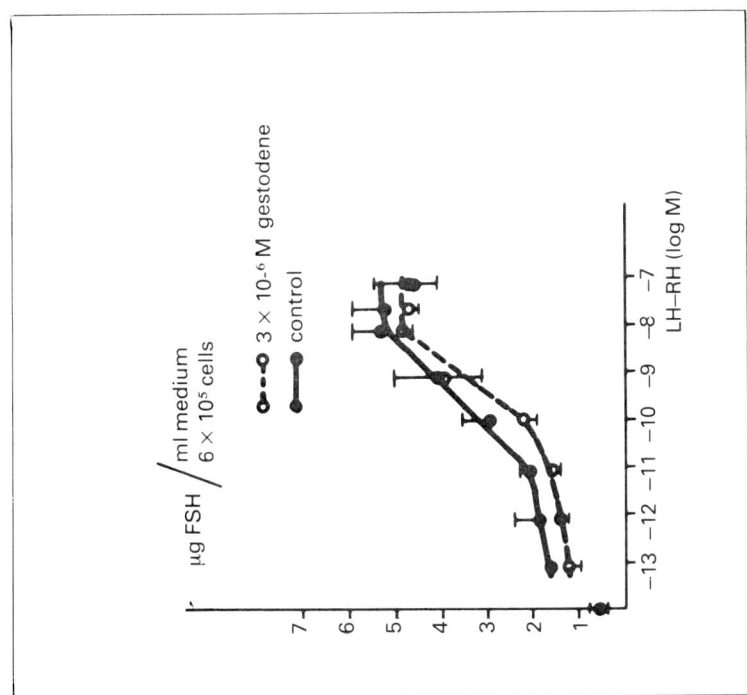

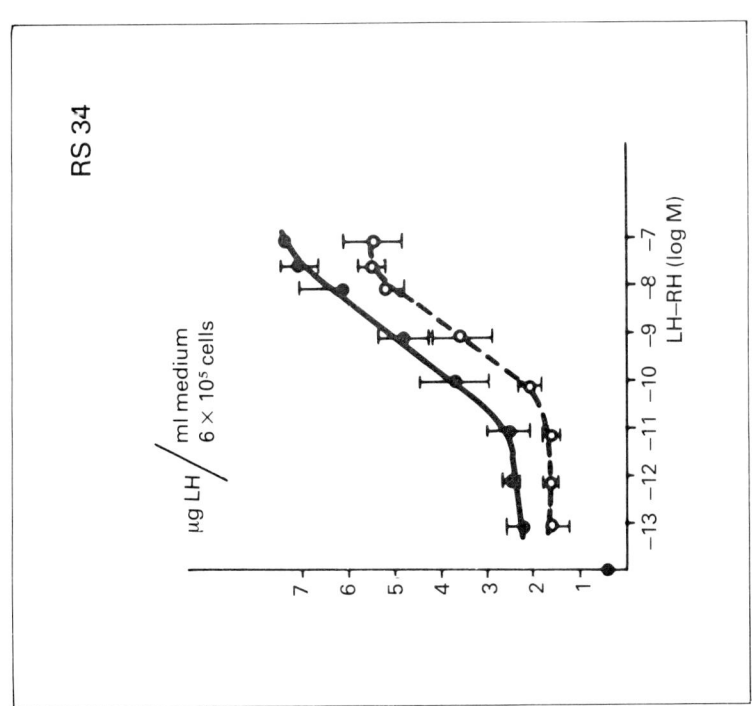

Figure 4   Modulation of LH and FSH release following stimulation by LH-RH in a primary cell culture of the pituitary front lobe

Ovulation inhibition with combination preparations

The functional parameters of the cycle under the effect of 75 μg of gestodene in combination with 30 μg of ethinyl estradiol administered daily over 21 days showed inhibition corresponding to an anovulatory cycle (Figure 5). The gestodene-containing combination not only brought a central inhibitory effect which led to an anovulatory cycle but also caused inhibition of cervical function and a reduction in the karyopyknotic index. The start of withdrawal bleeding occurred on an average 3 days after cessation of medication and the length and severity of bleeding, compared with the normal cycle, was decreased. It would appear of interest that no breakthrough bleeding was observed.

DISCUSSION

The present investigations show that the present trend towards reduction of the steroid dosage in oral contraceptives can be continued if biologically more active substances are available. The present study reveals that the minimum dosage[3] demanded by the WHO can be fulfilled by the use of a new progestogen which would keep possible side-effects as low as possible.

The present study succeeded in showing that gestodene can suppress the gonadotropin release stimulated by LH-RH. Suppression of the LH-RH induced LH release by progesterone has been found in women[7] and laboratory animals[8–11]. These results indicate that inhibition of ovulation caused by progestogens can be achieved at least partially by modulation of gonadotropin release at the level of the pituitary. They are supported by the findings presented. Moreover, experiments in this study suggest that gestodene exhibits greater biological activity than levonorgestrel with respect to its ability to alter gonadotropin release following stimulation by LH-RH. In the rat model described, gestodene would appear to be about three times more biologically effective than levonorgestrel. Higher biological activity of gestodene compared with levonorgestrel was also identified in the cell culture system. However, in this *in-vitro* system the differences between the two progestogens were not so marked as in the animal model.

These experimental data would suggest that a reduction in the dosage of progestogen in an oral contraceptive should be possible. This was revealed by examination of the limiting dosage for ovulation inhibition by gestodene. Daily administration of 40 μg of gestodene from the 5th to the 25th day of the cycle showed that in the case of 6 out of 7 test subjects inhibition of ovulation can be achieved. However, at this dosage follicle stimulation was observed in 4 of the 6 women studied.

It was also possible to demonstrate ovulation inhibition in a com-

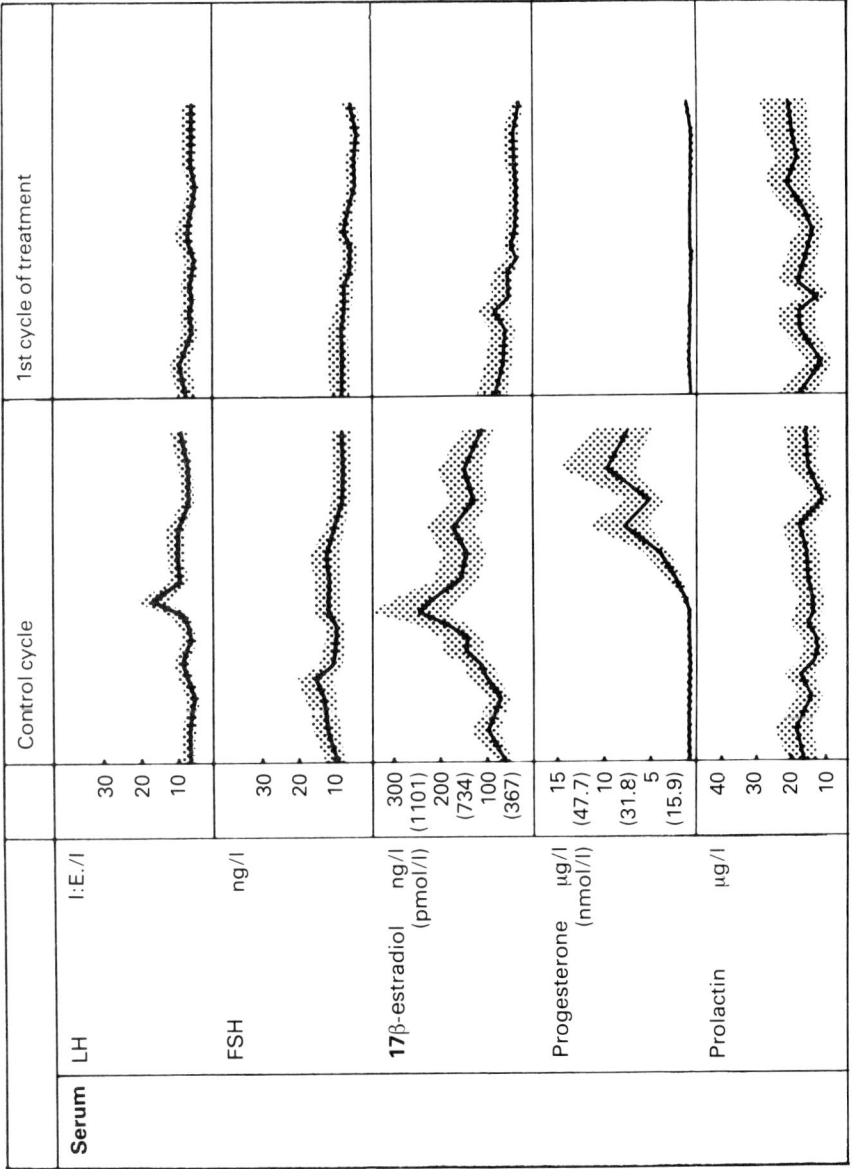

Figure 5   Behaviour of the hormone serum level in 10 subjects before and during administration of a daily dose of 75 μg of gestodene + 30 μg of ethinyl estradiol from the 5th to the 25th day of the cycle

bination preparation with 75 μg of gestodene + 30 μg of ethinyl estradiol.

Investigation into the androgenicity of gestodene showed that this substance exhibits similar properties with respect to the interaction with the androgen receptor as desogestrel. Moreover, it was possible in the present study to show that the biologically low androgenic activity of gestodene is similar to that of desogestrel. On the other hand, marked interaction of gestodene with the progestogen receptor was observed. It would also appear of importance that gestodene does not exhibit any interaction with the estrogen receptor.

The present results permit the conclusion to be drawn that gestodene is a new generation progestogen which can be used at lower dosages than progestogens used hitherto. The preconditions are thus provided for achieving a possible further reduction in side-effects.

REFERENCES

1. Lachnit-Fixson, U., Aydinlik, S. and Lehnert, J. (1984). Clinical comparison between a monophasic preparation and a triphasic preparation. In R. Rolland (ed.) *Advances in Fertility – Control and Treatment of Sterility*, pp 71–9. MTP Press Limited, Lancaster, Boston and The Hague.
2. Skouby, S. (1982). Laboratory and clinical assessment of a new progestational compound – desogestrel – a phase I study. *Acta Obstet. Gynecol. Scand. (Suppl.)*, 111–135.
3. World Health Organization (1978). Steroid contraception and risk of neoplasia. *WHO Tech. Rep. Ser.*, 619.
4. Spona, J. (1984). Androgenic properties of progestogens used in oral contraceptives. In R. Rolland (ed.) *Advances in Fertility – Control and Treatment of Sterility*, pp 89–98. MTP Press Limited, Lancaster, Boston and The Hague.
5. Brown, T. R., Bullock, L. and Bardin, C. W. (1979). *In vitro* and *in vivo* binding of progestins to the androgen receptor of mouse kidney: correlation with biological activities. *Endocrinology*, **105**, 1281–90.
6. Spona, J., Schneider, W. H. F., Bieglmayer, C., Schroeder, R. and Pirker, R. (1979). Ovulation inhibition with different doses of levonorgestrel and other progestogens: clinical and experimental investigation. *Acta Obstet. Gynecol. Scand. (Suppl.)*, **88**, 7–15.
7. Thompson, E. E., Arfania, I. and Taymor, M. L. (1973). Effects of estrogens and progesterone on pituitary response to stimulation by LHRH. *J. Clin. Endocrinol. Metab.*, **37**, 152–5.
8. Cumming, I. A., Buckmaster, J. M., Cerini, J. C., Cerini, M. E., Chamley, W. A., Findlay, J. K. and Goding, J. R. (1972). Effect of progesterone on the release of LH induced by a synthetic LH-RH in the ewe. *Neuroendocrinology*, **10**, 338–48.
9. Debeljuk, L., Arimura, A. and Schally, A. V. (1972). Effect of estradiol and progesterone on LH release induced by LH-RH in intact diestrous rats and anestrous ewes. *Proc. Soc. Exp. Biol. Med.*, **139**, 774–7.
10. Hilliard, J., Schally, A. V. and Sawyer, C. H. (1971). Progesterone blockade of the ovulatory response to intrapituitary infusion of LH-RH in rabbits. *Endocrinology*, **88**, 730–6.
11. Nakano, R., Kayashima, F., Kotsuji, F. and Tojo, S. (1974). Effect of gonadal steroids on the pituitary gonadotrophin response to LH-RH in the rat. *Endokrinologie*, **63**, 147–54.

4

Comparison of the effects of levonorgestrel and gestodene on pituitary gonadotropins, follicular development and cervical mucus

E. Eyong and M. Elstein

SUMMARY

The effect of two progestogens on cervical mucus, follicular develop-ment and the levels of follicle stimulating hormone (FSH), luteinizing hormone (LH) and progesterone in two groups of regularly men-struating women was analyzed.

During the administration of a 10-day course of $75\,\mu g$ gestodene and $75\,\mu g$ levonorgestrel, the serum LH, FSH and progesterone were depressed in all cases to levels incompatible with ovulation. Gestodene depressed the mean mid-cycle LH by 65% and FSH by 55%, while levonorgestrel depressed LH by 22% and FSH by 40%. Follicular maturation without rupture was present in 4 of the 5 patients who received levonorgestrel and in two patients who received gestodene. The estradiol and progesterone levels in the follicular fluid collected from one of these follicles were significantly lower than previously reported for normal preovulatory follicles. Cervical mucus was impen-etrable to sperm in both groups but the cervical score was more depressed in the gestodene than the levonorgestrel group (52% and 36% respectively).

These data collectively suggest that gestodene may be more potent than levonorgestrel, but further extension of the study is needed to confirm these preliminary findings.

INTRODUCTION

The search for lower dose progestogens capable of effectively inhibiting ovulation with fewer side-effects continues. Previous studies have shown that gestodene, a new progestogen, may be more potent in inhibiting ovulation than levonorgestrel[1]. The aim of this study is to compare the inhibitory effects of levonorgestrel and gestodene on pituitary gonadotropins, follicular development and cervical mucus.

SUBJECTS AND METHODS

This was a double-blind study of 15 regularly menstruating women (aged between 24 and 44 years) who elected for hysterectomy for benign gynecological disease (Table 1). Barrier contraception was required

Table 1   Indications for hysterectomy

Indications	Number of patients
Menorrhagia	8
Uterine fibroids and menorrhagia	6
Uterine prolapse	1

throughout the study for those liable to conceive and all hormonal contraception or steroid therapy was discontinued three months before the commencement of the trial.

The patients were randomly divided into 3 groups of 5 women, as follows:

(a)   Five women who received $75 \mu g$ gestodene daily for 10 days commencing on day 8 of the menstrual cycle.
(b)   Five women who received $75 \mu g$ levonorgestrel daily for 10 days commencing on day 8 of the menstrual cycle.
(c)   Five women who received no medication (for further mention of this group, see Chapter 5).

Groups a and b were investigated first for a control cycle and then for a treatment cycle as follows:

1. Ultrasound scanning
    Assessment of follicular development was carried out by examining patients in the supine position with a full bladder using the Diasonics DS1-RF sector real time scanner on cycles days 8, 10, 12, 14, 16, 18 and 21.
2. Venous blood was taken for assay of FSH, LH and progesterone on cycles days 8, 10, 12, 14, 16, 18 and 21.

3. Cervical score by Insler[2] and sperm penetration of mucus by Kremer[3] were quantified at mid-cycle (when the follicular diameter by ultrasound was about 16–18 mm) in the control cycle and on the same cycle day during the treatment cycle irrespective of the follicular size.
4. Hormone assay
   FSH and LH were measured by double antibody RIA[4].
   Progesterone (P) was measured by non-extraction double antibody RIA employing danazol as protein binding blocking agent[5].

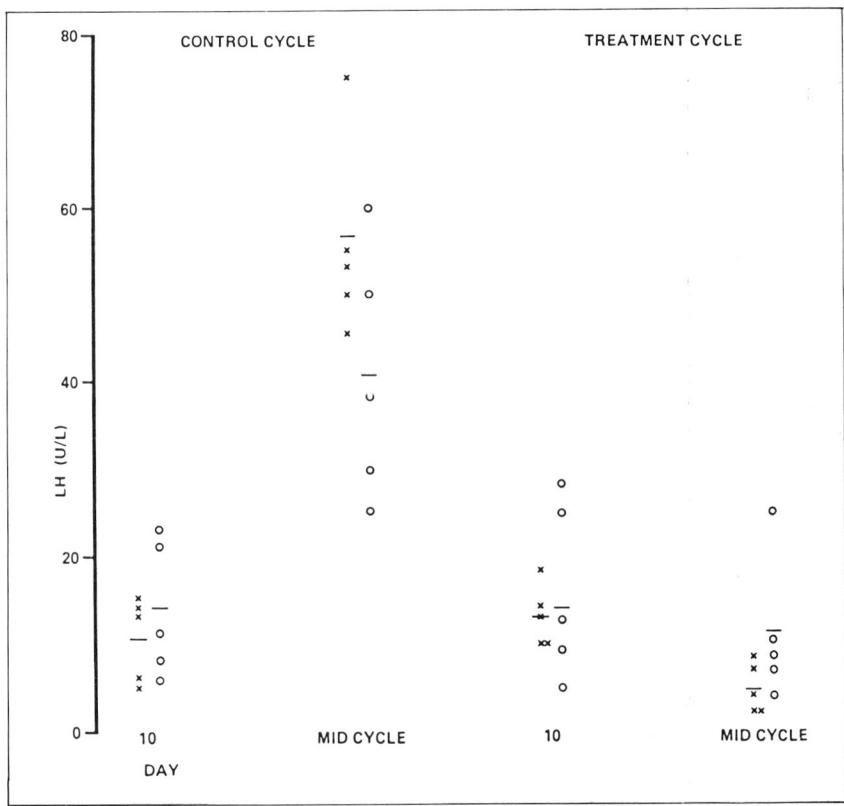

Figure 1   Serum LH levels in the control and treatment cycles of subjects who received a 10-day course of either levonorgestrel or gestodene
x = gestodene-treated subjects
o = levonorgestrel-treated subjects
— = mean LH values (*n* = 5 in each group)

After the course of treatment hysterectomy was performed on all patients (day 19–21 of the menstrual cycle) and the biochemical and histological effects of these progestogens on the endometrium were investigated (see Chapters 5 and 6).

RESULTS

All subjects recruited for the study ovulated in the control cycle, with the preovulatory follicular diameter ranging between 18 and 23 mm. Ovulation was inhibited in the treatment cycle in all subjects, irrespective of the progestogen ingested. The mid-cycle plasma LH values were suppressed by 65% with gestodene, and by 22% with levonor-

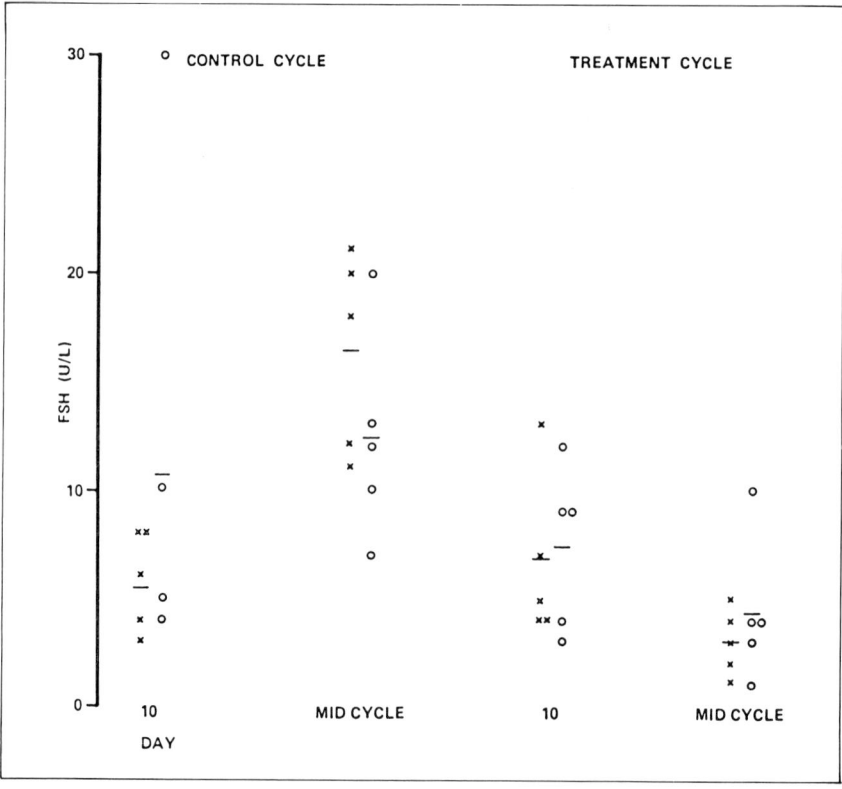

Figure 2   Serum FSH levels in the control and treatment cycles of subjects who received a 10-day course of either levonorgestrel or gestodene
x = gestodene-treated subjects
o = levonorgestrel-treated subjects
— = mean FSH values ($n = 5$ in each group)

gestrel, below the early follicular phase levels during the treatment cycle (Figure 1). The FSH levels fell by 55% with gestodene and by 40% with levonorgestrel (Figure 2). Due to the small number of subjects studied the results were not subjected to any statistical tests of significance. Progesterone values were significantly inhibited in all subjects below 2 nmol/1, irrespective of the progestogen ingested.

Follicular maturation

Follicular maturation without rupture was demonstrated in both treatment groups. With gestodene, 2 patients had follicular maturation, while with levonorgestrel 4 patients (i.e., twice the number) had follicular maturation. Follicles with a diameter of 30 mm were present to the time of surgery (Figure 3). We aspirated 12 ml of follicular fluid from one of these follicles and obtained the following steroid levels:

Estradiol – 202 ng/ml (normal level: 616–3662 ng/ml)
Progesterone – 280 ng/ml (normal level: 1068–18058 ng/ml)[6].

Cervical score

In the control cycle all subjects had a satisfactory cervical score (Table 2). In the treatment cycle the mean cervical score fell by 52% with gestodene and by 36% with levonorgestrel.

Table 2   Cervical score in patients on levonorgestrel and gestodene

| | Levonorgestrel | | Gestodene | |
Patient	Control cycle	Treatment cycle	Control cycle	Treatment cycle
1	11	4	12	8
2	11	11	12	8
3	12	10	12	5
4	12	10	12	4
5	12	3	12	4

Sperm penetration (Table 3)

As with the cervical score, satisfactory sperm penetration of mucus was recorded in all subjects in the control cycle. There was, however, no significant sperm penetration of the mucus in both groups in the treatment cycle, although the mucus was thicker, more opaque and impenetrable to sperm with gestodene.

Table 3 Sperm penetration test (total height = 5 cm) on the cervical mucus of patients treated with levonorgestrel and gestodene.
Number of sperm refers to the number seen in the lower power field of the microscope

Patient	Levonorgestrel				Gestodene			
	Control cycle		Treatment cycle		Control cycle		Treatment cycle	
	Number of sperm	Height of penetration (cm/h)	Number of sperm	Height of penetration (cm/h)	Number of sperm	Height of penetration (cm/h)	Number of sperm	Height of penetration (cm/h)
1	>200	5	10	0.5	>100	5	<10	2
2	>200	5	<5	1	>500	5	<5	0.1
3	>50	2	0	0	>200	5	0	0
4	>200	5	<10	0.2	>400	5	0	0
5	>100	5	0	0	>100	5	<10	0

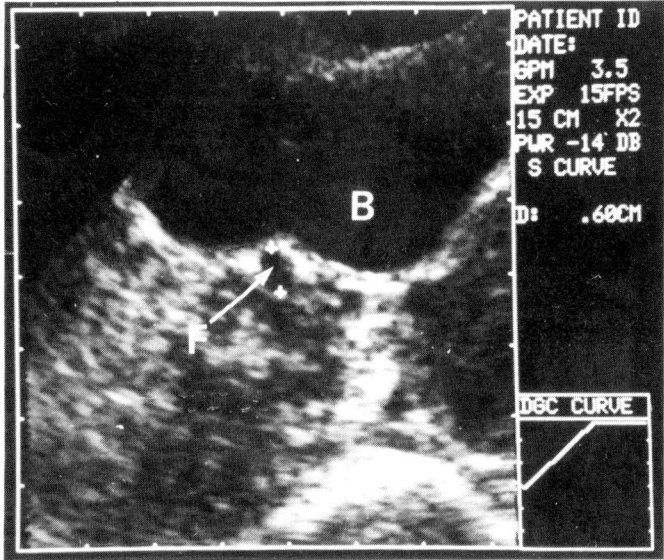

Figure 3.1 Cycle day 8. The left ovary demonstrated a developing follicle with an average diameter of 6 mm

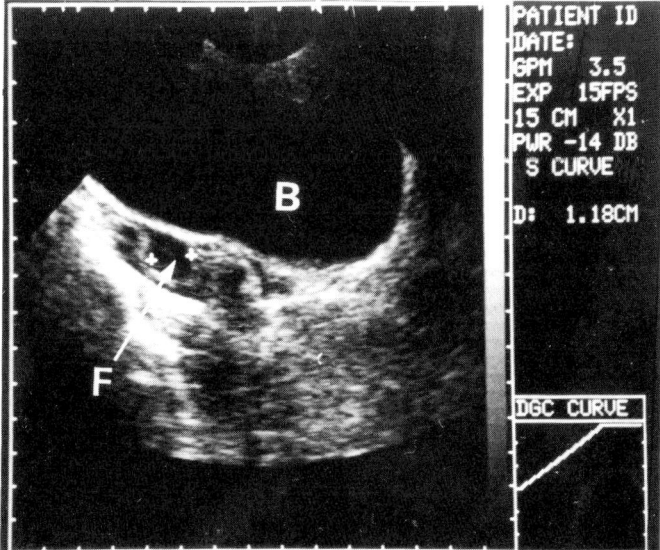

Figure 3.2 Cycle day 12. The follicle has increased in size to an average diameter of 12 mm

Figure 3 Sagittal sections through the left ovary of a subject demonstrating follicular maturation without rupture during the administration of 75 μg of levonorgestrel for 10 days, commencing on day 8 of the menstrual cycle.
U = uterus, F = follicle and B = bladder

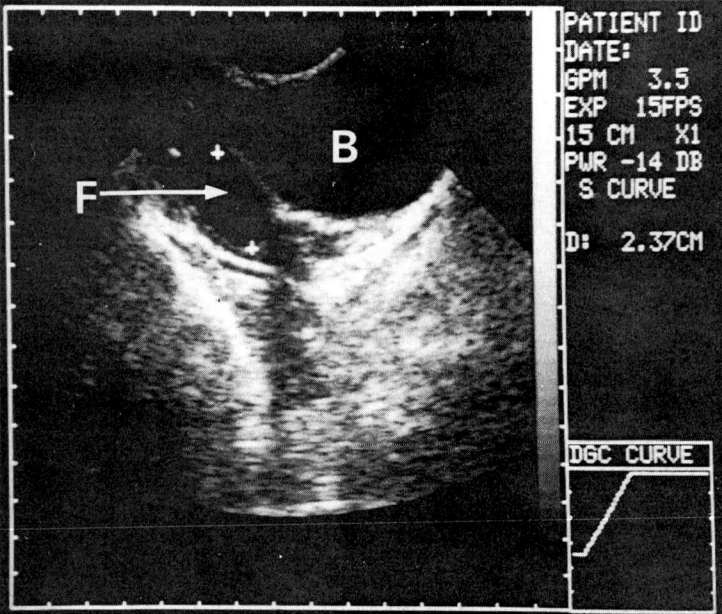

Figure 3.3   Cycle day 16. The follicle is even bigger, with an average diameter of 24 mm

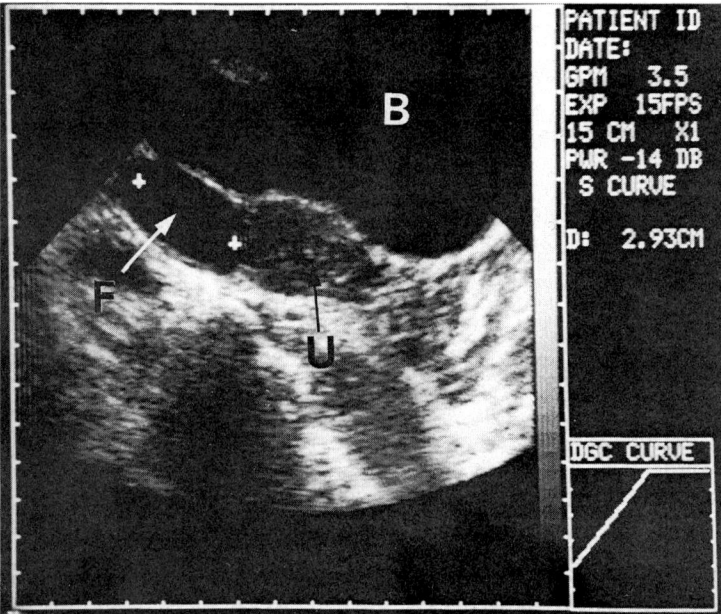

Figure 3.4   Cycle day 20. A day prior to hysterectomy, the follicle now has an average diameter of 30 mm

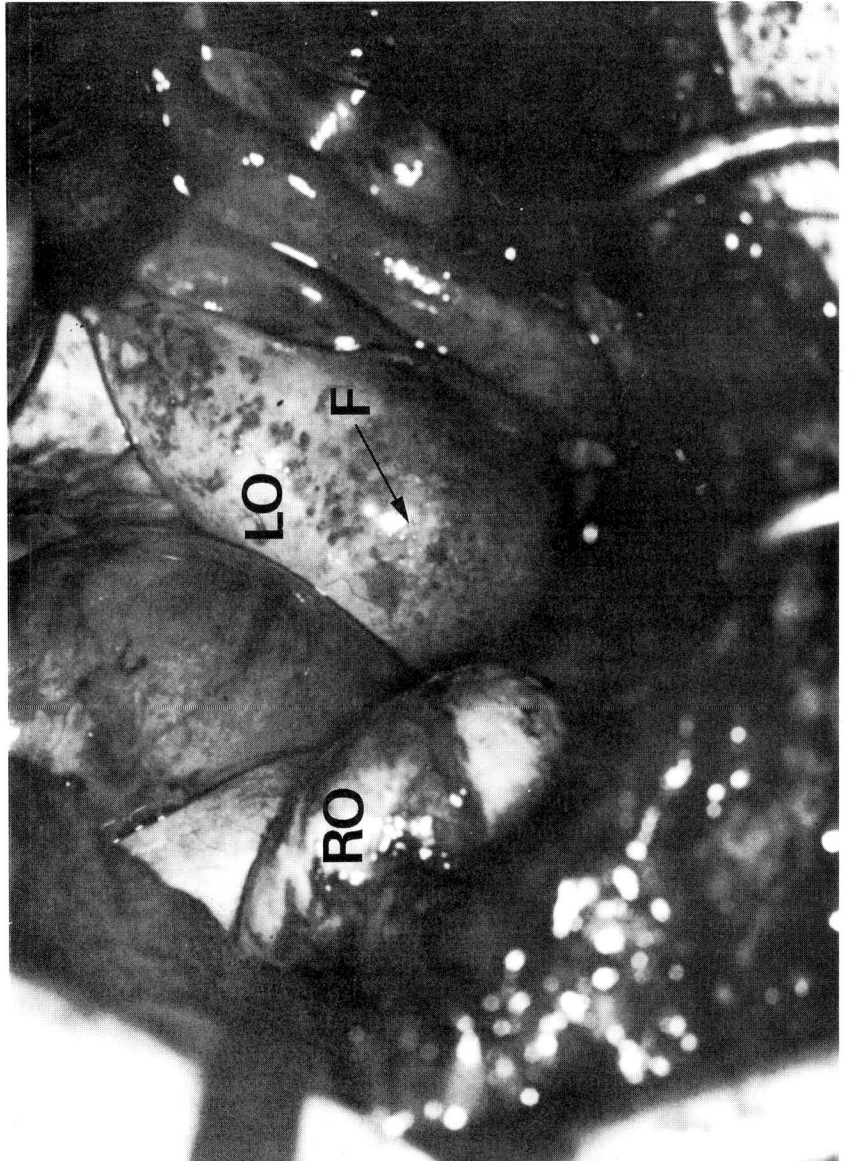

Figure 3.5   Cycle day 21. At operation the right ovary (RO) and left ovary (LO) are shown. Note the size of the left ovary due to the follicle (F). The uterus is not shown. Follicular fluid (12 ml) was aspirated from it for steroid estimation

DISCUSSION

The results obtained in this study show no evidence of a gonadotropin peak suggestive of ovulation with the administration of either gestodene or levonorgestrel to subjects. Gestodene would, however, appear to be more potent (thrice) than levonorgestrel in suppressing the mid-cycle LH surge (65% and 22% respectively, Figure 1). Similar results with gestodene and levonorgestrel have been reported in the past[1]. The FSH levels were equally suppressed by gestodene and levonorgestrel (55% and 40% respectively, Figure 2).

The preovulatory follicular diameter obtained by ultrasound in this trial is consistent with previous reports[7]. There was ultrasonic evidence of follicular maturation without rupture (Figure 3) in 2 gestodene subjects and 4 levonorgestrel subjects (twice the number).

Failure of follicles to rupture was evidenced by their persistence until the time of surgery (cycle days 19–23) and the low levels of serum progesterone. The demonstration of follicular maturation during progestogen ingestion in this trial confirms previous reports that FSH and LH suppression does not necessarily inhibit follicular maturation[8]. In fact it has been recently suggested that lack of FSH suppression may be an explanation for follicular maturation[9]. Follicular maturation would have been higher with levonorgestrel, as both FSH and LH were suppressed to a lesser extent than with gestodene. The estradiol and progesterone levels in the follicular fluid from one of these follicles were significantly lower than previously reported for normal follicles.

As with previous reports[10-13], both progestogens made the cervical mucus unfavourable and impenetrable to sperm. Gestodene depressed the cervical score by 52% of the control cycle, while levonorgestrel depressed it by 36%. Although there was no significant sperm penetration in either group, the mucus appeared thicker, more opaque and, therefore, impenetrable to sperm with gestodene, again suggesting its potency might be greater than that of levonorgestrel.

CONCLUSION

From the results obtained in our study it would appear that gestodene is likely to show more potent biological activity than levonorgestrel. Although the numbers studied were small and the results obtained could therefore not be subjected to statistical tests of significance, the data obtained in this study do suggest that gestodene might be superior to levonorgestrel in inhibiting pituitary gonadotropins and follicular development and making cervical mucus impenetrable to sperm.

REFERENCES

1. Spona, J., Schneider, W. H.F., Bieglmayer, Ch., Schroeder, R. and Pirker, R. (1979). Ovulation inhibition with different doses of levonorgestrel and other progestogens. Clinical and experimental investigation. *Acta Obstet. Gynecol. Scand. (Suppl.)*, **88**, 7–15.
2. Insler, V., Melmed, H., Eichenbrenner, I., Serr, D. and Lunnerfeld, D. (1972). The cervical score. *Int. J. Gynecol. Obstet.*, **10**, 223–8.
3. Kremer, J. A. (1965). A simple sperm penetration test. *Int. J. Fertil.*, **10**, 209–15.
4. Ferguson, K. M., Hayes, M. and Jeffcoate, S. L. (1982). A standardised multicentre procedure for plasma gonadotrophin radio-immunoassay. *Ann. Clin. Biochem.*, **19**, 358–61.
5. Ratcliffe, W. A., Corrie, J. E. J., Dalziel, A. and Macpherson, J. S. (1982). Direct ^{125}I-radioligant assays for serum progesterone compared with assays involving extraction of serum. *Clin. Chem.*, **28**, 1314–18.
6. Fowler, R. E., Chan, S. T. H., Walters, D. E., Edwards, R. G. and Steptoe, P. C. (1977). Steroidogenesis in human follicles approaching ovulation as judged from assays of follicular fluid. *J. Endocrin.*, **72**, 259–71.
7. Hackeloer, B. J., Fleming, R., Robinson, H. H., Adam, A. H. and Coutts, J. R. T. (1979). Correlation of ultrasonic and endocrinologic assessment of human follicular development. *Am. J. Obstet. Gynecol.*, **135**, 122–8.
8. Bergquist, C. and Lindgren, P. G. (1983). Ultrasonic measurement of ovarian follicles during chronic LRH agonist treatment for contraception. *Contraception*, **28**, 125–33.
9. Tafurt, A. C., Sobreville, L. A. and De Estrada, R. (1980). Effects of progestin-oestrogen combination and progestational contraceptives on pituitary gonadotrophins, gonadal steroids and sex hormone binding globulin. *Fertil. Steril.*, **33**, 261–6.
10. Elstein, M., Briston, P. G., Hewitt, K. J., Kirk, D. and Miller, H. (1976). The effect of daily norethisterone (0.35 mg) on cervical mucus and on urinary LH, pregnanediol and oestrogen levels. *Br. J. Obstet. Gynaecol.*, **83**, 165–8.
11. Kesseru-Koos, E. (1971). Influence of various hormonal contraceptions on sperm migration *in vivo*. *Fertil. Steril.*, **22**, 584–603.
12. Ulstein, M. and Myklebust, R. (1982). Ultrastructure of cervical mucus and sperm penetration during use of triphasic oral contraceptive. *Acta Obstet. Gynecol. Scand. (Suppl.)* **105**, 45–9.
13. Zanartu, J., Pupkin, M., Rosenberg, D., Guenero, R., Rodriguez-Bravo, A. and Puga, J. (1968). Effect of oral continuous progestogen therapy in microdose on human ovary and sperm transport. *Br. Med. J.*, **7**, 263–6.

5

Endometrial receptor response to two progestogens, levonorgestrel and gestodene

E. N. Chantler, R. Sharma, E. Eyong and M. Elstein

The object of this trial is to compare uterine biochemical variables which are gestodene-sensitive, in women who have received 10 days' therapy with either levonorgestrel or gestodene. One of the main effects of oral progestogens is the suppression of gonadotropin release by the anterior pituitary. However, both the absence of gonadotropin-stimulated production of ovarian steroids and the action of the progestogens on steroid receptors affect the uterus. Such uterine responses to oral steroids have been used in the past to attempt to quantify the relative potency of different progestogens. In the interpretation of such results it is important to remember that the response relates to a particular biochemical variable and should not be extended to a comparison of the whole body response to a particular progestogen.

In this study we chose two progestogen-sensitive systems in the endometrium, firstly the level of the nuclear estradiol receptor and secondly the activity of the enzyme estradiol dehydrogenase, which converts estradiol to estrone in response to progesterone or progestogens. At this stage only the receptor data are available.

METHODS

Women were chosen for inclusion in this study who fulfilled the following criteria:

(a) No malignant gynecological disease.
(b) Not using oral contraception or IUDs.
(c) No steroid therapy during the preceding 3 months.
(d) No contra-indication for progestogens.

Three study regimes were compared:

(1) Five women who had taken 75 µg gestodene daily for 10 days from day 8 of the menstrual cycle (i.e., when all Graafian follicles were less than 10 mm in diameter).

(2) Five women who had taken 75 µg levonorgestrel daily for 10 days from day 8 of the menstrual cycle.

(3) Five women who had had no treatment.

All the women underwent hysterectomy after the completion of these regimes, i.e., 19–23 days after the beginning of the last menstrual bleeding.

The majority of the endometrium was removed by scraping, immediately the uterus was removed, and plunged into liquid nitrogen. Upon processing the endometrium was homogenized at 0°C in 10 mM Tris/HCl buffer pH 7.4 containing 0.5 mM dithiothreitol and 10% v/v glycerol, and centrifuged at 800 g for 10 min. The pellet was repeatedly washed and recentrifuged and finally passed through a 400 mesh stainless steel grid to remove tissue fragments. The purity of the preparation was checked microscopically using phase contrast. Samples of the nuclear pellet were frozen in liquid nitrogen and disrupted by 15 seconds treatment with a dismembrator. The resultant powder was resuspended in buffer and incubated at 4°C for 12 hours with 5 nM [2, 4, 6, 7-³H]-estradiol (92 Ci/µmol) with or without 0.2 µM diethylstilbestrol. The sample was then mixed with 0.17 g hydroxyapatite (HAP) for 30 min, the HAP was separated by centrifugation and washed 4 times in the Tris buffer at 4°C. Finally the radiolabelled steroid was extracted from the HAP with 1.0 ml absolute ethanol; 4.0 ml Optiphase scintillant (Fisons, UK) was added and the steroid was estimated by liquid scintillation counting. The DNA content of the sample was measured fluorimetrically using m-diaminobenzoic acid[1].

RESULTS

The procedures adopted were chosen to give a stable nuclear preparation, uncontaminated with cytosolic components. These criteria were not always obtained by us using some of the methods described in the literature. Incubation at 4°C under conditions reported to allow measurement of the available or unoccupied receptors gave a stable level of receptor under saturating conditions.

At this stage of the study the levels of available receptor shown in Table 1 have been found:

Table 1

Treatment	Mean level of receptor pmol E_2/mg DNA	SD	Range
Control n = 4	0.55	0.38	0.142–0.897
Levonorgestrel n = 4	1.29	0.77	0.665–2.55
Gestodene n = 3	2.91	0.83	2.08–3.88

INTERPRETATION

The techniques for the examination of nuclear estrogen receptors presented some unexpected problems. Microscopic analysis of nuclear preparations made using published methods which had previously been used in this Department showed frequent contamination with cytosolic components. Furthermore, the buffer/detergent mixtures used slowly degraded the nuclear envelope, resulting in loss of the receptor. The procedure adopted gave preparations which were uncontaminated with tissue fragments (by microscopic examination). In addition, the receptor was released from the nuclei by homogenization and bound to HAP, prior to measurement; this procedure afforded a consistent reliable assay. The saturation of the nuclear binding sites with [³H] estradiol at 4°C measures available receptor sites which are implicated in the nuclear expression of the steroid[2].

The results of this study are preliminary and the small number of women studied to date does not allow a statistically valid comparison to be made. However, as the mean levels of receptors in the study groups are separated by a standard deviation, obvious trends in the data can be seen. Both of the progestogens studied increase the level of available nuclear receptors but to a different extent. Gestodene treatment results in a 530% increase in the receptor concentration compared to the control, whilst levonorgestrel produced a 235% increase. Thus, at comparable concentrations gestodene doubles the concentration of available nuclear estrogen receptors.

The physiological significance of the proportion of available/total nuclear estrogen receptor sites is unclear, as the distinction is based upon their relative thermal stability. Moreover, it is not known whether unoccupied sites are active in the potential expression of estrogens by receptors.

Some explanations of our results can be made using the classical theory of receptors which is based on the translocation of the activated receptor from the cytosol to the nuclear compartment, activation of the appropriate genome and return of the unoccupied receptor to the cytosol. The synthesis of the estrogen receptor is known to be inhibited by progesterone and its derivatives; in addition, the binding of estradiol to the cytoplasmic receptor is also inhibited[3]. Thus the expected result of progestogen therapy, in the absence of estrogens, would be a depletion of the *total* nuclear estrogen receptor level. Our study is restricted to the *available* receptors, which appear to increase under these conditions. This may result from either:

(a) A decrease in the binding affinity of estradiol to the receptor, in the presence of the progestogens, without altering its rate of entry into the nucleus, or

(b) A prolonged residence of the unoccupied receptor in the nucleus after dissociation of the estrogen.

A different analysis may be made using data which suggest an alternative to the classic theory, in which both unoccupied and occupied receptors normally reside in the nucleus and the presence of a cytosol receptor may be a preparative artefact[4,5]. In this case the observed progestogen-mediated inhibition of estrogen binding to the receptor which occurs in the cytosol[3] may under carefully controlled conditions occur in the nucleus. This would result in an increase in the proportion of unoccupied receptor sites in the nucleus as a response to progestogens.

The presence of such unoccupied estrogen receptors in the nucleus could arise from either:

(a) Low levels of estradiol in the endometrium, as a result of suppression of ovarian steroid synthesis (by the progestogen),

(b) An inability of the receptor to bind estradiol within the nucleus, or

(c) Retention of the unoccupied receptor within the nuclear compartment.

In each of these cases the result would be a reduced ability of the endometrium to respond to estradiol, and these data indicate that this effect would be expected to be greater in gestodene treatment than with levonorgestrel. Thus gestodene may be expected to be superior to levonorgestrel in its suppression of the estrogenic proliferation of the endometrium, with obvious contraceptive advantages. However, the significance of parallel influences such as the hormonal output by the relative predominance of the ovarian follicles in the gestodene subjects might play an important role.

An alternative measurement of the nuclear action of the progestogens may be obtained by measuring the levels of estradiol dehydrogenase, which is elevated by progestogens, resulting in an inhibition of estradiol action[6]. We are currently investigating this system.

REFERENCES

1. Vytasek, R. (1982). *Anal. Biochem.*, **120**, 243–8.
2. Fleming, H. and Gurpide, E. (1980). *J. Steroid Biochem.*, **13**, 3–11.
3. Di Carlo, E., Reboani, C., Conti, G., Portaleone, P., Viano, L. and Genazzani, E. (1980). In E. Genazzani, F. Di Carlo and W. I. P. Mainwaring (eds) *Pharmacological Modulation of Steroid Action*, pp 61–74. Raven Press, New York.
4. King, W. J. and Greene, G. (1984). *Nature*, **307**, 745–7.
5. Welshons, W. V., Lieberman, M. E. and Gorski, J. (1984). *Nature*, **307**, 747–9.
6. King, R. J. B., Whitehead, M. I., Campbell, S. and Minardi, J. (1978). *Postgrad. Med. J.*, **54** (Suppl. 2), 65–8.

6

Comparative histology of the endometrium under treatment with levonorgestrel and gestodene

N. Y. Haboubi, E. Eyong, E. N. Chantler and M. Elstein

SUMMARY

The histological changes of the endometrium in two groups of patients (one treated with gestodene for 10 days, and the other treated with levonorgestrel for 10 days) were assessed blindly. A third group of untreated patients was used as a control. It was found that:

(1) The control 'untreated' group can be differentiated easily from the two treated groups.
(2) No single parameter can differentiate clearly between the two treated groups.
(3) Using groups of parameters, the gestodene-treated patients have more thin-walled dilated vessels, stromal edema and total impairment of ciliogenesis.

INTRODUCTION

The progestogen component of the combined oral contraceptive pill produces side-effects which are dose-related. This has prompted a search for new progestogenic agents which can maintain an adequate contraceptive effect on the reproductive organs when administered in a lower dose.

This study is concerned with comparing the effect of the well known and potent progestogen levonorgestrel and the new agent gestodene on the endometrial histology.

MATERIALS AND METHODS

Three groups of randomly allocated patients were used for histological assessment. These were as follows –

1st group: gestodene-treated – 75 µg per day for 10 days starting
        day 8
2nd group: levonorgestrel-treated – 75 µg per day for 10 days start-
        ing day 8
3rd group: untreated

The pathologist was unaware which patient belonged to which
group. To achieve maximum preservation of the endometrial
histology, the gynecologist who performed the hysterectomies made a
Y-shaped incision on one side of each uterus, through the wall and
into the endometrial cavity, leaving the other wall intact (Figure 1).
A small amount of cotton wool was placed in these incisions and then
the specimen was put in formalin and sent to the laboratory.

A total of 14 such uteri were received, identified only by name. The
specimens were left in the fixative for 24 hours and then examined
and cut. An average of 8 blocks was taken from each uterine cavity.

For histological assessment only sections with intact surface epithelium were scrutinized. The following parameters were used:

(1) *Glandular shape* was small and uniform or dilated and tortuous.
(2) *Glandular secretory activity* was judged by the type of cells, irres-
    pective of presence or absence of secretory vacuoles. The typical
    secretory cells have round and vesicular nuclei with fine chroma-
    tin and sometimes prominent nucleoli.
(3) *Glandular proliferative activity* was judged by the presence of basa-
    lis-type cells which have high N/C ratio, elongated dense nuclei
    and inconspicuous nucleoli, together with frequent mitoses and
    nuclear pseudostratifications.
(4) *Stromal cells.* Only non-granulocytic cells were looked for, and
    they were categorized into
    (a) Spindle cells with scanty indistinct cytoplasm and dense oval
        nuclei. These are typically seen in the proliferative phase.
    (b) Plump cells with more cytoplasm and vesicular nuclei as
        typically seen in the secretory phase.
(5) *Development of spiral arterioles* was looked for specifically in the
    middle third of the endometrium where they are more abundant
    and easily recognized. Poorly developed arterioles were thin elon-
    gated vascular structures with no cuffing (Figure 2). The well
    developed arterioles are tortuous and have abundant peri-
    vascular cuffing (Figure 3).
(6) *Endometrial thickness* was measured by graticulated eye piece.
(7) *Thin walled dilated vessels* were measured semiquantitatively.
    These vessels were histologically similar to peliosis hepatis and
    mostly seen beneath the surface epithelium (Figure 4).

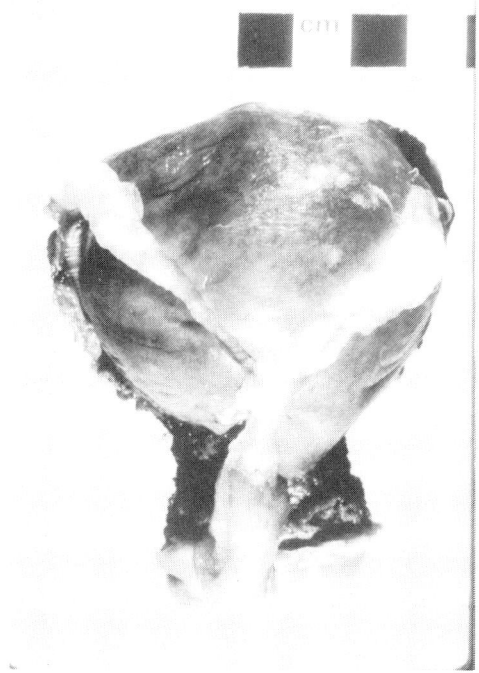

Figure 1   The Y-shaped incision on one side of the uterus is loosely packed with cotton wool

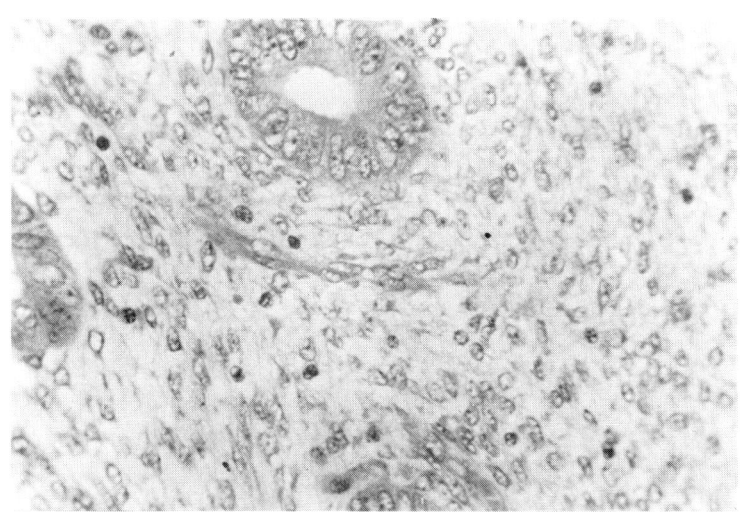

Figure 2   Thin and collapsed 'undeveloped' spiral arterioles

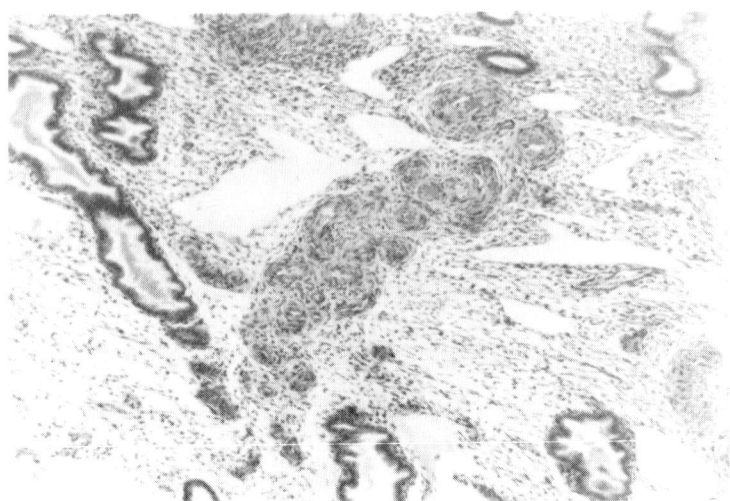

Figure 3   Well developed, tortuous spiral arterioles

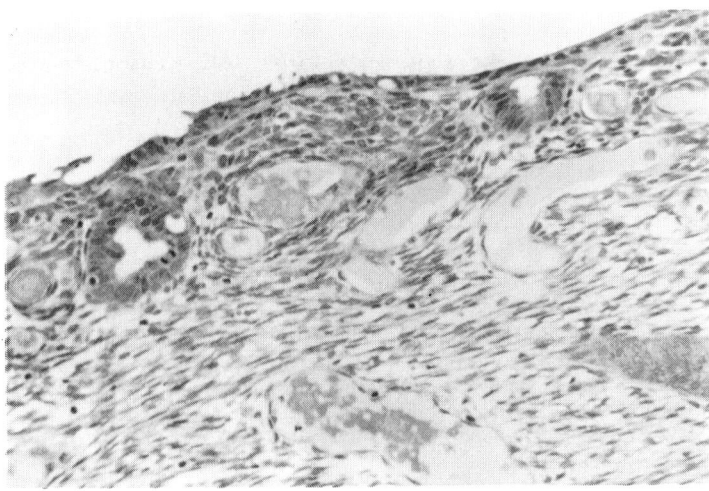

Figure 4   Large number of thin dilated vessels situated mostly beneath the surface epithelium

(8) *Stromal edema* was measured semiquantitatively.
(9) *Stromal hemosiderin* was measured semiquantitatively.
(10) *Ciliated cells* were located in the first 10 glands examined. They have characteristic rounded cells with matching vesicular nuclei. In three specimens PTAH/iron hematoxylin was employed to spot those cells but it was found that they could be identified by simple hematoxylin and eosin staining. They were scored as:
> 5 or more cells/10 glands is normal.
> 1–5 cells/10 glands is reduced.
> No cells/10 glands is impaired.
(11) *Ciliogenesis* was looked at in the same 10 glands as above and was scored semiquantitatively.

RESULTS

The results of the 14 patients were scored on a single chart (Table 1). It appeared that 5 patients had normal secretory endometrium, and when the code was broken these were the control group.

When the data were analyzed critically (Table 2) in the 2 treated groups:

(1) It was found that no single parameter we used can differentiate clearly between the levonorgestrel and the gestodene patients.
(2) It was noted, however, that using a group of parameters significant differences can be seen, as follows:

(a) Four out of 4 patients treated with gestodene have thin dilated ectatic vessels, while 2 out of 5 have that in the levonorgestrel group.
(b) Stromal edema was found in 3 out of 4 patients in the gestodene group and 1 out of 5 in the levonorgestrel group.
(c) Ciliogenesis was impaired in all gestodene patients but found to be normal in 2 out of 5 patients treated with levonorgestrel.

DISCUSSION

It is obvious from this pilot study that both drugs have produced significant changes in the endometrium to such an extent that it made it easy to differentiate them from the control group.

However, it is important to note that the changes in the two treated groups show more similarities than differences, but it must be remembered that the patients underwent one cycle treatment and it is possible that giving the drugs for more than one cycle can produce even more delineating results.

Table 1

PATIENT	PB	MD	RD	MC	JL	KW	PD	BM	PA	MM	PS	MA	BH	EB
Gland shape	small uniform	coiled	small uniform	coiled	small uniform	mixed	small uniform	coiled	mixed	coiled	small uniform	coiled	mixed	mixed
Glandular secretory activity	−	+++	−	+++	−	+	−	+++	+	+++	−	+++	++	++
Glandular proliferative activity	+	−	++	−	+	+	+	−	+	−	−	−	+	+
Stromal cells	Spindle compact	Plump	Plump	Plump & early predecid	Plump & spindle	Plump & spindle	Spindle compact	Plump	Plump	Plump	Spindle compact	Plump	Plump & spindle	Plump & spindle
Development of spiral arteries	−	+	−	++	+	+	−	++	++	++	+	++	++	++
Thin-walled vessels	+++	−	+	−	+	−	++	−	−	−	−	−	++	+
Endometrial thickness in cms	0.15	0.4	0.2	0.35	0.1	0.2	0.1	0.3	0.2	0.35	0.15	0.4	0.25	0.15
Stromal edema	−	++	+	+++	+	−	−	−	−	++	−	++	++	+
Stromal hemosiderin	++	−	++	−	−	−	+	−	−	−	+	−	+	+
Ciliated cells	N	N	−	N	→	→	N	N	−	N	N	N	−	−
Ciliogenesis	−	N	−	N	−	−	N	N	−	N	N	N	−	−

Table 2

LEVONORGESTREL					PATIENT	GESTODENE			
MS	PA	KW	PD	EB		PB	BH	RD	JL
Small & uniform	Mixed	Mixed	Small & uniform	Mixed	Gland shape	Small & uniform	Mixed	Small & uniform	Small & uniform
—	+	+	—	++	Glandular secretory activity	—	++	—	—
—	+	+	+	+	Glandular proliferative activity	+	+	++	+
Spindle	Plump	Plump & spindle	Spindle & compact	Plump & spindle	Stromal cells	Spindle & compact	Plump & spindle	Plump	Plump & spindle
+	++	+	—	++	Development of spiral arteries	—	++	—	+
—	—	—	++	+	Thin walled vessels	+++	++	+	+
0.15	0.2	0.2	0.1	0.15	Endometrial thickness cms	0.15	0.25	0.2	0.1
—	—	—	—	+	Stromal edema	—	+	+	+
+	—	—	+	+	Stromal hemosiderin	++	+	++	—
N	—	↓	N	—	Ciliated cells	N	—	—	↓
N	—	—	N	—	Ciliogenesis	—	—	—	—

7

Clinical investigations with a new gestodene-containing oral contraceptive (Femodene®)

R. Unger

Various clinical studies have been carried out with the gestodene combination preparation consisting of $75 \mu g$ of gestodene and $30 \mu g$ of ethinyl estradiol. Since the ovulation inhibition studies and the results of metabolism and hemostasis studies will be reported elsewhere, this presentation will deal with only Phase II and Phase III clinical studies. The test preparation is to be launched in Great Britain under the name Femodene. In all other countries it will probably be marketed under names such as Gynera®, Femovan®, Ginoden®, and the like.

PHASE II CLINICAL STUDY

In the Phase II clinical study the cycle control and tolerance of 2 different-dose test preparations, namely, a combination of $75 \mu g$ of gestodene + $30 \mu g$ of ethinyl estradiol (Femodene) and $100 \mu g$ of gestodene + $20 \mu g$ of ethinyl estradiol (preparation A) were compared over 6 cycles with the time-proven widely marketed preparation Microgynon® (= $150 \mu g$ of levonorgestrel and $30 \mu g$ of ethinyl estradiol). The aim of the investigations was to demonstrate whether one of the 2 test preparations was superior to the commercial product.

The study was carried out at 21 test centres in 5 European countries, the various preparations being randomly allocated to the test subjects. When the volunteers were recruited for the study, care was taken that the usual contra-indications to oral contraceptive use were taken into account.

A total of 561 women took part in the study, of whom 540 were included in the evaluation. This means that there were 176 women in the Femodene cohort, 179 in the cohort given the alternative test preparation and 185 in the Microgynon cohort (Table 1).

It can be seen from Table 2 that in the Femodene cohort 93.2% of

Table 1   Numbers of cases per preparation

	1	2	3	Total
Evaluable	176	179	185	540
Not evaluable	10	3	8	21
Total	186	182	193	561

1 = Femodene®
2 = Preparation A
3 = Microgynon®

the women completed the study over 6 cycles, in the alternative cohort 85.5% and in the Microgynon cohort 86%. Thus data are available on 1022, 1015 and 1055 treatment cycles respectively.

Although the volunteers admitted medication errors in 50 cycles, no pregnancies occurred during the treatment period. The course of the cycles was normal with all 3 preparations during treatment, i.e., in the vast majority of cases the cycle length was 26–30 days, the duration of bleeding 4–7 days, and the amount of flow was classified as 'normal'. As expected, the percentage of cases of scant bleeding increased but it did not reach the level usually found with the high-dose preparations.

The absence of withdrawal bleeding was also relatively rare in all 3 cohorts. In the Femodene cohort there were 2 cases of absent withdrawal bleeding over 1 cycle and in another volunteer no withdrawal bleeding occurred over 2 cycles. On the other hand, in the other 2 cohorts there were 12 and 6 cases of absent withdrawal bleeding respectively over 1 cycle. Thus the incidence of absent withdrawal bleeding in the 3 cohorts amounted to 0.4% for Femodene, 1.2% for the alternative preparation and 0.6% for Microgynon.

In accordance with usual definitions, irregular bleeding during use of the preparations was subdivided into the categories: spotting, break-

Table 2   Duration of therapy

	Femodene ®	Preparation A	Microgynon ®
Cycle 1	1.1%	0%	1.1%
Cycle 2	0%	3.4%	0.5%
Cycle 3	2.8%	2.8%	4.3%
Cycle 4	2.3%	2.8%	1.1%
Cycle 5	0.6%	5.6%	7.0%
Cycle 6	93.2%	85.5%	86.0%
Total number of cycles	1022	1015	1055

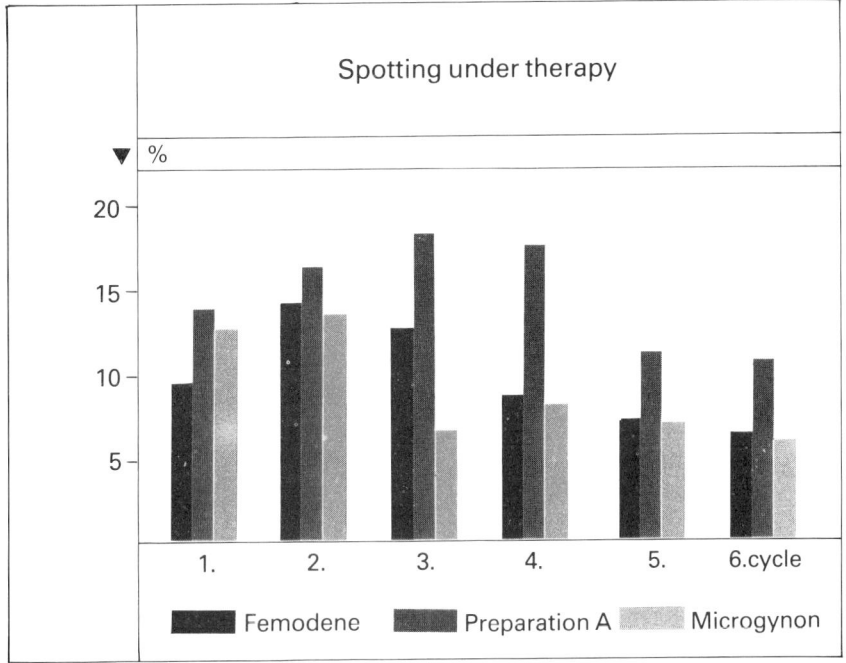

Figure 1   Spotting while under therapy

through bleeding, and spotting and breakthrough bleeding in the same cycle, during treatment. Ignoring medication errors and whether or not irregular bleeding had already been mentioned in the case history, the picture shown in Figure 1 was evident.

As Figure 1 shows, in the Femodene cohort an initial increase in spotting is followed by a progressive decrease. There is no essential difference between the Femodene and Microgynon cohorts. Gestodene performs better in the 1st cycle and Microgynon in the 3rd cycle. It is particularly clear how badly the test preparation which only contains 20 μg of ethinyl estradiol performs. Once again, we have confirmation of experience that lowering the ethinyl estradiol concentration to below 30 μg results in an unacceptable bleeding pattern.

Considering the breakthrough bleeding from the same angle, two things are obvious. Firstly, there is the very low incidence of breakthrough bleeding during treatment with Femodene and, secondly, the marked inferiority in this respect of the test preparation which contains 20 μg of ethinyl estradiol (Figure 2).

Based on the total number of cycles, breakthrough bleeding has an incidence of 1.8% during treatment with Femodene and 3.1% during treatment with Microgynon.

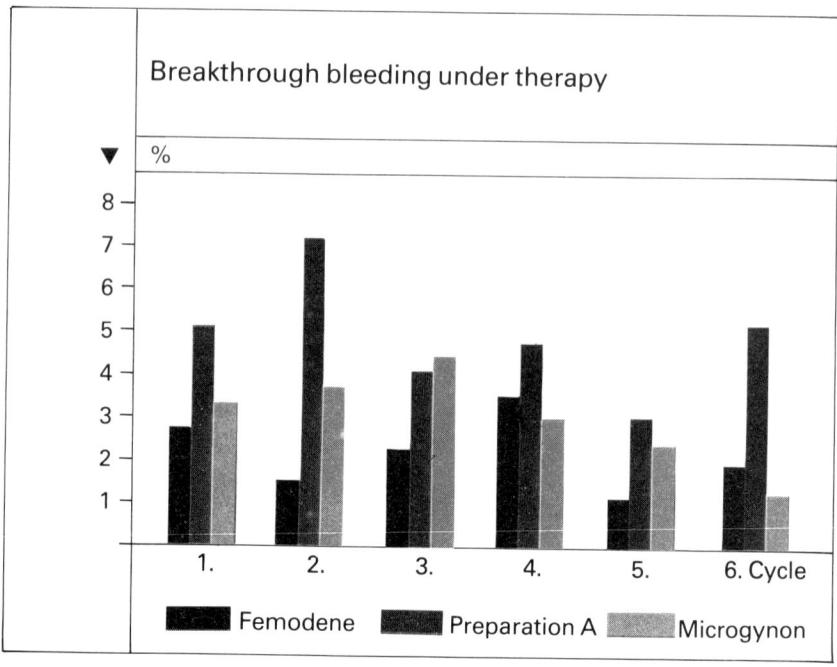

Figure 2   Breakthrough bleeding while under therapy

Owing to the poor performance by the alternative test preparation A subsequent data obtained with this combination are not reported, since further development of the product was abandoned.

To assess the tolerance of an oral contraceptive, subjective and objective side-effects need to be identified. Subjective side-effects are not dealt with here, since the number of cases is too small to draw conclusions. I would just like to say that there are seldom differences between the Femodene and Microgynon cohorts as regards individual symptoms.

Objective side-effects

Objective side-effects occurred in only a few cases. Serious side-effects such as thrombophlebitis or hepatopathy were not observed at all.

To assess *changes in weight*, the values determined in the 6th treatment cycle are compared with the baseline values. In 86.9% of the cases, weight was practically unaffected during treatment with Femodene. In the remaining women, weight gains of more than 2 kg were markedly more frequent than weight losses. Changes in weight were similar for the Microgynon cohort.

To assess *changes in blood pressure*, comparisons are also made with the baseline values. Since, as expected, in all groups studied systolic blood pressure is subject to greater fluctuations than diastolic blood pressure, the latter will be considered in more detail.

As an example, in the 6th treatment cycle of women in the Femodene cohort the changes in diastolic blood pressure shown in Table 3 were observed. Out of a total of 161 women, 143 (= 88.8%) came into the 'normal category' with unchanged values of below 90 mm Hg. There were 5 cases of increased blood pressure compared with 7 cases in which previously elevated values became normal. One woman, whose blood pressure rose to more than 105 mm Hg, was admitted to hospital after stopping the medication. No cause was found. However, the blood

Table 3 Diastolic blood pressure in Femodene patients before the start of therapy and in cycle 6

| Before start of therapy | Cycle 6 | | | |
	Below 90 mm Hg	90-105 mm Hg	Above 105 mm Hg	Total number of women
Below 90 mm Hg	143	4	1	148
90–105 mm Hg	7	6	0	13
Above 105 mm Hg	0	0	0	0
Total number of women	150	10	1	161

pressure remained high and unstable even without medication, so that there does not seem to be a causal association between that and the test preparation.

The values for Microgynon and also for the other cycles appeared almost identical.

Treatment was stopped prematurely because of side-effects in the case of 5.7% of the Femodene cohort. Irregular bleeding was stated as the reason for this in 3 cases. The other symptoms were only mentioned by 1 woman in each case.

PHASE III CLINICAL STUDY

The clinical Phase II study was followed immediately by clinical Phase III in which there was no control group. The maximum duration was 24 cycles. The study was designed so that at least 200 women could be treated over the *full* 24 cycles, in order to meet the requirements of various regulatory authorities.

Thirty-one test centres in 6 European countries were involved in the study, in which clinics and established gynecologists participated.

To evaluate the results, the cycles of the Phase III clinical study and the Femodene cycles of the Phase II study were combined. The following data were obtained:

Altogether 707 women were treated, so we have a general view of 9947 treatment cycles. Although the volunteers admitted medication errors in 184 cycles, no pregnancies occurred.

The *bleeding pattern* during treatment with Femodene can be seen in Table 4. As expected, irregular bleeding during treatment was observed more frequently in cycles in which medication errors occurred. There is an increase in spotting from 6.5% to 28.8%, and in breakthrough bleeding from 0.7% to 4.4%.

Based on all treatment cycles, the incidence of spotting is 6.9%, of breakthrough bleeding 0.8% and of spotting and breakthrough bleeding 0.7%.

Table 4   Intermenstrual bleeding with and without intake error

	Spotting	BTB	Spotting and BTB	Total number of cycles
No tablets omitted	6.5%	0.7%	0.7%	9668
Tablets omitted	28.8%	4.4%	0 %	184

The distribution of irregular bleeding in individual cycles is shown in Table 5. It is common knowledge that irregular bleeding decreases with increasing length of treatment.

Withdrawal bleeding was absent during medication in a total of 59 out of 9947 cycles, i.e., the incidence of absent withdrawal bleeding amounted to 0.6%.

If we consider the tolerance of the test preparation Femodene the *body weight* remains practically unaffected with no change after the

Table 5   Intermenstrual bleeding

	Spotting	BTB	Spotting and BTB in same cycle
Before	4.7	0.6	1.6
Cycle 1	9.9	1.8	0.9
Cycle 3	8.5	0.8	1.0
Cycle 6	5.5	1.0	1.4
Cycle 12	5.8	0.5	0.7
Cycle 18	5.1	0.3	1.4
Cycle 24	4.6	0	0

All data in %

3rd cycle in 97.1% of all women, and with no change after the 24th cycle in 80.5% of all women.

The *blood pressure* values exhibited the following picture: In the case of systolic blood pressure, on an average 98.5% of the values were considered to be 'normal', both before and after treatment. In the case of diastolic blood pressure the figure was 94.7%. These percentages are hardly subject to variation during the test period (Table 6).

Table 6   Normal blood pressure under therapy

Cycle 3	Systolic	596 out of 608 women = 98.0%
	Diastolic	573 out of 607 women = 94.4%
Cycle 6	Systolic	617 out of 632 women = 97.6%
	Diastolic	591 out of 631 women = 93.7%
Cycle 12	Systolic	393 out of 396 women = 99.2%
	Diastolic	380 out of 396 women = 96.0%
Cycle 18	Systolic	271 out of 273 women = 99.3%
	Diastolic	260 out of 273 women = 95.2%
Cycle 24	Systolic	206 out of 209 women = 98.6%
	Diastolic	197 out of 209 women = 94.3%

The diastolic blood pressure in the 6th treatment cycle is again taken as an example here (Table 7). Blood pressure was normal before and after treatment in 591 women (= 96.6%). There were 13 cases of deterioration, in contrast with 17 cases in which previously high blood pressure improved. The 1 case in which blood pressure reached values above 105 mm Hg has already been reported in the analysis of the Phase II study. There was a second case involving a young woman who was very much overweight and in whom the values suddenly increased to 170/120 in the 6th treatment cycle. The blood pressure

Table 7   Diastolic blood pressure in Femodene patients before the start of therapy and in cycle 6

	Cycle 6			
Before start of therapy	*Below 90 mm Hg*	*90–105 mm Hg*	*Above 105 mm Hg*	*Total number of women*
Below 90 mm Hg	591	11	2	604
90–105 mm Hg	17	10	0	27
Above 105 mm Hg	0	0	0	0
Total number of women	608	21	2	631

was normal both before and after. The supervising physician did not regard this as a reason to stop therapy but instead advised the woman to lose weight. Thus the value measured in the 6th cycle should be interpreted as a unique observation.

Women whose blood pressure before treatment was in the limit range between 90 and 105 mm Hg showed improvement relatively frequently during treatment, the values becoming normal. By the 3rd cycle, in 15 out of 25 cases (= 60%) of previously high blood pressure the values had become normal.

Subjective side-effects (Table 8)

As is the case with all ovulation inhibitors, here too the favourable effect on dysmenorrhea is striking. There was a slight increase in the number of cases of decreased libido during therapy. In the case of all other symptoms lower values than the baseline ones were reached at the latest after the 6th cycle, and normally before. The 3 most frequently mentioned subjective side-effects were breast tension, headache and nervousness.

Table 8   Subjective side-effects

	Before	1	3	Cycle 6	12	24
Dysmenorrhea						
slight	23.5	16.2	7.6	5.7	5.8	2.3
severe	6.6	0	0	0	0	0
Nausea	2.7	11.6	5.6	0.9	0.7	0
Vomiting	0.1	0.3	0.3	0	0	0
Dizziness	3.4	3.0	2.0	2.1	1.9	0.5
Breast tension	8.6	13.2	9.0	7.4	9.6	7.3
Varicose disorders	1.7	1.6	1.7	2.5	1.4	0.9
Headache	9.0	10.9	9.0	6.6	7.2	6.4
migrainous	1.0	0.7	0.9	0.8	1.7	0.5
Nervousness	8.9	10.1	9.1	8.1	7.4	7.8
Depression	2.1	2.3	1.6	1.8	2.4	0.9
Increased libido	0	0.9	1.2	0.6	2.2	0.5
Decreased libido	1.6	2.3	3.3	3.5	5.3	5.0

All data in %

Objective side-effects

As regards objective side-effects, acne and edema decreased during therapy. One woman in each case mentioned these side-effects as a reason for dropping out of the study.

In 1 woman (= 0.1%) thrombosis occurred in the 3rd cycle. This superficial thrombosis, which lasted 2 weeks, was so slight that the supervising physician did not regard it as a reason to stop therapy. It did not occur again during further treatment.

Two women (0.2%) mentioned the symptom 'hepatopathy'. In 1 case no conclusion can be drawn because the patient failed to visit the supervising physician again. In the other case, after specific questioning it transpired that the patient merely had 'a short attack of liver pain'.

The drop-out rate due to side-effects amounted to 12%, or 85 women out of the total study population, which is within the range normally observed in a study of this type. The most frequently mentioned reasons were spotting and breakthrough bleeding, each of which was stated by just 3% of all women.

CONCLUSION

Based on the available data, the following summary can be given: Femodene can be considered to be a further development in the field of monophasic ovulation inhibitors. Its good cycle control, resulting in cycle stability, and its good tolerance may well increase the acceptability of low-dose oral contraceptives.

8

Interim results of a UK study comparing a new monophasic pill containing gestodene to Microgynon 30® and proceeding to open assessment

R. J. Kirkman

This paper reports the results up to June 1985 of Phase II and III clinical trials of the formulation Femodene – i.e., 21 tablets of $75\,\mu g$ gestodene and $30\,\mu g$ ethinyl estradiol.

The aims of the study were:

(1) To compare the contraceptive efficiency, cycle control and side-effects of Femodene with that of a well established low-dose pill, Microgynon 30, over 6 cycles.

(2) To assess the long-term acceptability of Femodene.

METHOD

Thirty-four centres and individual doctors in the United Kingdom took part (Table 1), using a study population of women aged 16–35 years. Our protocol specified the usual oral contraceptive contra-indications, precautions and reasons for stopping medication, and in addition excluded women with amenorrhea, undiagnosed abnormal vaginal bleeding, a diastolic blood pressure over 90 mm Hg or who were breast feeding. We therefore recruited a mixture of some women who were already taking oral contraceptives and some without prior medication.

The 6-cycle comparison was carried out double-blind, so that neither the doctor nor the patient knew whether they were allocated the well-established Microgynon or the 'new' pill. Randomization was in blocks of 10. After 6 cycles all patients took Femodene for a further 12 cycles, but still without breaking the original randomization code.

Admission protocol included a brief history, and a physical exam-

Table 1

Centre	Doctor		Centre		Doctor
Bar Hill	R. A. Newsom	GP	London	FP	H. M. Freeman
Bingley	S. M. Richardson	FPC	Luton	FPC	S. Smith
Birmingham	J. A. Dewsbury	FPC	Middlesbrough	GP	B. Levie
Bournemouth	G. A. Langsdale	GP	Newbury	GP	M. E. Youdan
Bracknell	B. J. Ranscombe	GP	Newcastle-upon-Tyne	FPC	D. Tacchi
Burgess Hill	P. Bye	FPC	Newport (Gwent)	GP	M. Mehrotra
Chorley	F. W. Yates	GP	Sheffield	FPC	M. Griffiths, P. Heathcote, H. King R. Kirkman, Nandasoma & M. Staniforth
Crawley	P. Stillman	GP			
Edinburgh	E. Barden & N. B. Loudon	FPC	Sheffield	FPC	J. Wordsworth
Edinburgh	A. R. Milne	GP	South Darenth	GP	J. A. Nicholson
Farnborough	G. R. Caird & R. E. Hamill	GP	Southend	GP	U. R. Hutter & C. A. V. Goodchild
Hessel	P. J. Miller	GP	Southend	GP	A. R. W. Bowring & D. E. Pelta
Hull	M. S. Setiya	GP	South Queensferry	GP	J. D. Stuart
Hull	N. A. M. Somerville	GP	Steyning	GP	A. Frank
Hyde	S. Davies	GP	Stoneyburn	GP	P. Chima
Leicester	S. Finlay & R. Ellis	GP	Tonbridge	GP	P. Cunningham
London	S. H. Houghton	FPC	Twyford	GP	P. Thomas
			Windsor	GP	C. B. Butcher

GP = General practitioner. FPC = Family Planning Clinic

ination including breast palpation, vaginal examination and cervical smear. Patients kept a daily record of pill-taking and vaginal bleeding (i.e., loss heavy enough to require sanitary protection) and/or spotting (i.e., loss not heavy enough to require protection) and were reviewed every 3 months.

At each follow-up visit we recorded the patient's weight, blood pressure, menstrual pattern including spotting, bleeding, dysmenorrhea and objective symptoms such as acne, chloasma, edema, thrombophlebitis or hepatopathy. The patients were then asked a general question about their health and any symptoms spontaneously reported (e.g., headache, nausea) were recorded. Completed diary cards were returned with follow-up forms to Schering Health Care for analysis.

A withdrawal bleed was regarded as any period of continuous bleeding which occurs in the tablet-free period. Cycle length was taken as the time from the start of 1 cyclical bleed up to but not including, the 1st day of the next withdrawal bleed.

COMPARISON OF FEMODENE WITH MICROGYNON 30

Up to June 1985, 374 women (Table 2) had either completed the first 6 cycles or dropped out during that period. Patients still progressing through this phase have not been included in this analysis.

Table 2   Patient recruitment and randomization

	Femodene	Microgynon 30	Total
Number recruited	202	199	401
Number analyzed	189	185	374
Number of cycles	1062	1034	2094

Admission data

Age distribution was similar between the 2 groups, but with slightly more young subjects in the Femodene group (Figure 1). All but 6 were Caucasian. The 2 groups were fairly well balanced regarding the number of pregnancies or abortions (Table 3). 59% of the Femodene group and 52% of the Microgynon group were nulliparous.

There was no significant difference, on admission, between the 2 treatment groups in menstrual regularity, duration and intensity of flow, dysmenorrhea or occurrence of intermenstrual bleeding. Table 4 shows contraceptive use within the 3 months prior to recruitment. 53% of patients had been using combined oral contraceptive preparations and 31% had been using no contraception.

Table 3   Obstetric history

Number of pregnancies	Number and percentage of patients	
	Femodene	Microgynon 30
None	105 (59%)	92 (52%)
1	32 (18%)	33 (19%)
2	26 (15%)	30 (17%)
3	12 (7%)	15 (9%)
4 or more	3 (1%)	6 (3%)
Total	178	176

Table 4   Previous contraceptive history

Primary contraceptive method	Number (and percentage) of patients	
	Femodene	Microgynon 30
None	51 (27%)	64 (35%)
Combined oral contraceptives	110 (58%)	94 (51%)
'Mini-pills'	8 (4%)	2 (1%)
IUD	3 (2%)	7 (4%)
Other	17 (9%)	18 (9%)
Totals	189	185

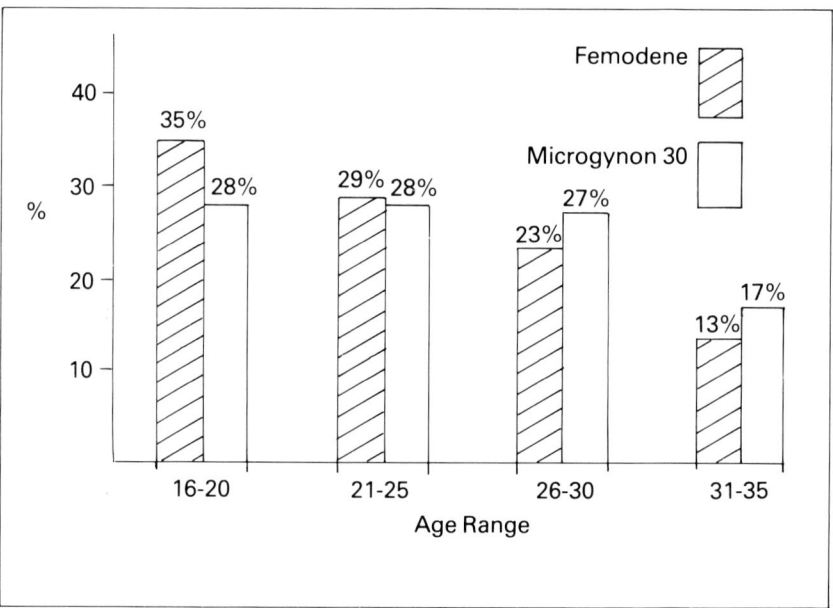

Figure 1   Age distribution

Results

Of the 374 patients who entered the study, 320 (86%) completed 6 cycles. Data were collected from 1062 cycles in the Femodene group and 1034 cycles in the Microgynon group. Only 8 patients (4 from each group) were lost to follow-up (Table 5).

Table 5   Number of patients

Completed cycle	Number (and percentage) of patients			
	Femodene		Microgynon 30	
1	189	(100%)	185	(100%)
2	186	(98%)	183	(99%)
3	184	(97%)	179	(97%)
4	172	(91%)	169	(91%)
5	167	(88%)	162	(88%)
6	164	(87%)	156	(84%)
Total number of cycles	1062		1034	

Withdrawals from the study

The rate of patient withdrawal was similar in both treatment groups (Figure 2), with a total loss of approximately 15% of patients recruited.

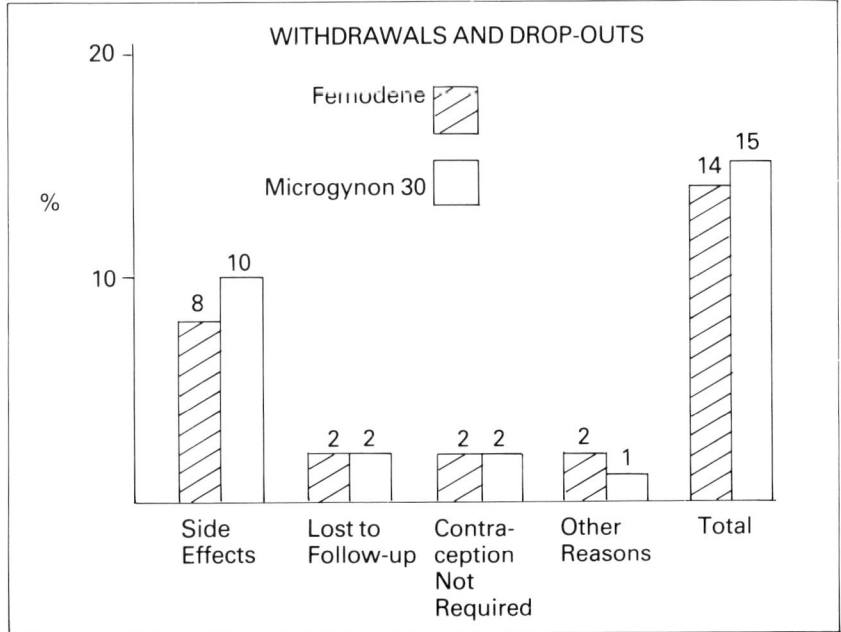

Figure 2   Withdrawals and drop-outs

Unacceptable side-effects caused withdrawal of 8% of Femodene and 10% of Microgynon 30 patients.

No pregnancies occurred during this phase despite tablet omissions in 71 Femodene cycles and 80 Microgynon cycles.

Cycle control was good in both groups, but with slightly more long or short cycles in the Microgynon group.

Withdrawal bleeding was between 4 and 7 days in the great majority of patients in both treatment groups and there was no difference in this regard to duration or intensity of bleeding, incidence of absent withdrawal bleeding or amount of dysmenorrhea, whether looked at overall, or categorized into subgroups according to the pretreatment history.

There were statistically significant differences between the 2 preparations regarding data on intermenstrual bleeding. Breakthrough bleeding (with or without spotting) occurred in 28% of patients in the Microgynon group compared to 17% in the Femodene group (1% significance $X^2 = 6.770$, df) (Figure 3). The numbers reporting spotting

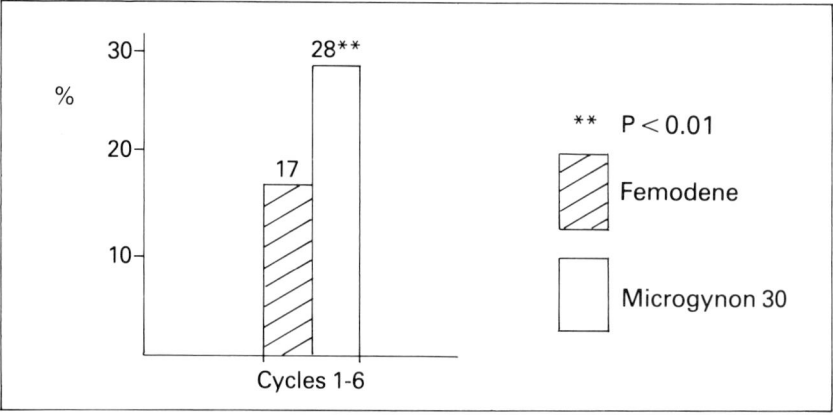

Figure 3   Intermenstrual bleeding (percent patients reporting)

only were similar in each treatment group and the incidence of both spotting and breakthrough bleeding was higher in the 1st 3 cycles than in the 2nd 3.

Looking at the total number of cycles observed, the incidence of all 3 categories of intermenstrual bleeding was significantly higher in the Microgynon group (0.1% significance $X^2 = 15.007$, df) (Figure 4).

Figure 5 illustrates also the quicker control of cycles achieved by Femodene in that intermenstrual bleeding in this group returned to pretreatment levels by the 3rd cycle, whereas it fell more slowly over all 6 cycles in the patients taking Microgynon.

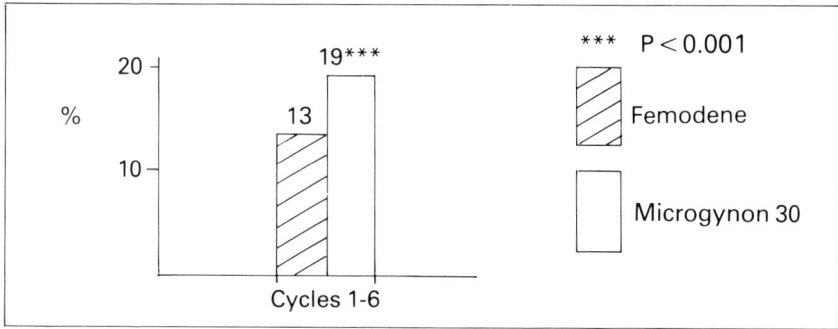

Figure 4   Intermenstrual bleeding cycle incidence

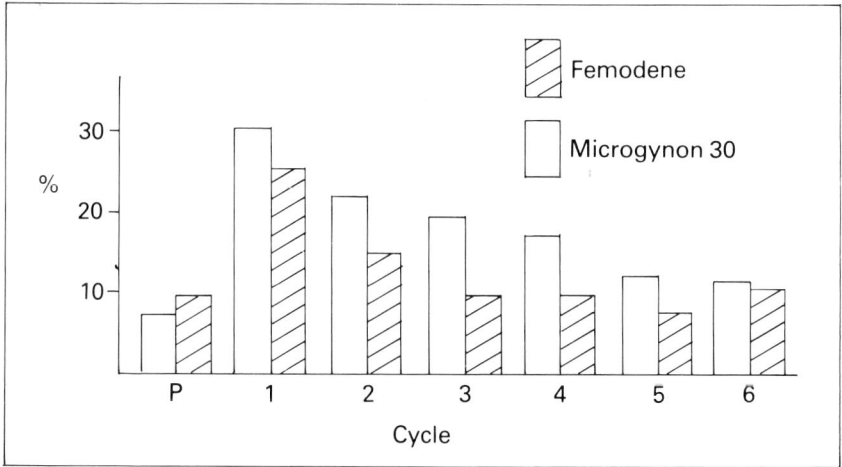

Figure 5   Intermenstrual bleeding

The incidence of intermenstrual bleeding was higher in cycles in which tablets were missed, but patient numbers were not sufficient to draw conclusions.

We found that the subgroups of patients who had been using combined oral contraceptives prior to entering the study showed less intermenstrual bleeding than the patient subgroups who had not (Figure 6). In those patients previously using oral contraceptives and switching to Femodene there tended to be a higher incidence of spotting over the 1st 3 cycles, but a slightly lower incidence of breakthrough bleeding. In patients switching to Microgynon 30, however, there was an increase in both spotting and breakthrough bleeding which was slow to decline. In patients who had not previously been using oral contraceptives the increase in intermenstrual bleeding was again more

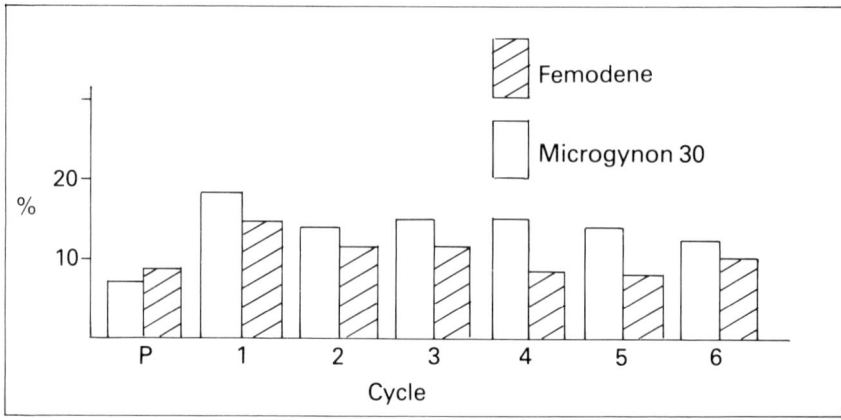

Figure 6   Intermenstrual bleeding in previous oral contraceptive users

persistent in the Microgynon group than in the Femodene group and the proportion of breakthrough bleeding to spotting was higher (Figure 7). There was no significant difference between the 2 preparations in other physical parameters.

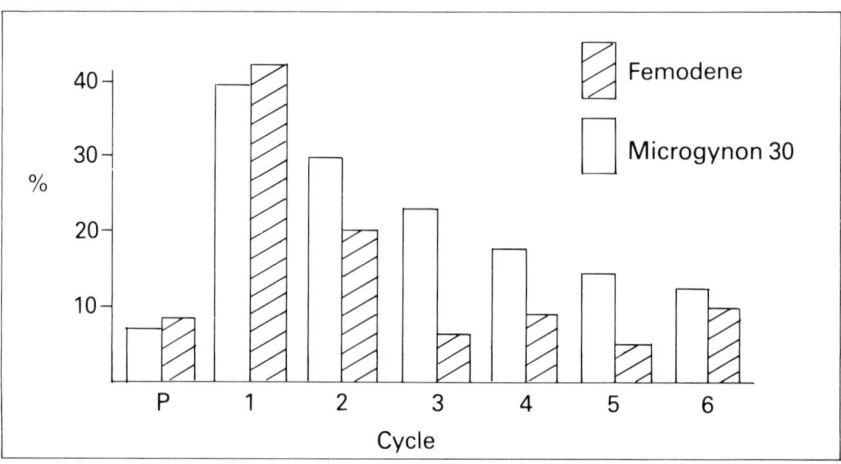

Figure 7   Intermenstrual bleeding in new patients

Hypertension defined as systolic over 140 mm Hg and diastolic over 90 mm Hg was reported on only 4 occasions in women taking Femodene and 2 occasions in women taking Microgynon.

Body weight changes are shown in Table 6. 66% of the Femodene group and 62% of the Microgynon group remained within a fluctuation of ± 2 kg.

Table 6 Body weight changes after 6 months

| | Number (and percentage) of patients | |
	Femodene	Microgynon 30
Loss > 2 kg	25 (16%)	19 (13%)
Loss (2–0.5) kg	33 (21%)	25 (17%)
Constant ± 0.5 kg	40 (26%)	34 (24%)
Gain (0.5–2) kg	29 (19%)	31 (21%)
Gain > 2 kg	28 (18%)	37 (25%)
Totals	155	146

Side-effects

Of the objective side-effects (Table 7) the most common was acne, which was reported for 6% of patients in the Femodene group and 5% in the Microgynon group. The incidence did not vary with time. Edema was present in 6 Microgynon patients (3%) and 1 Femodene patient.

Chloasma was noted for 1 Femodene patient and for 2 Microgynon patients. Thrombophlebitis and hepatopathy were not observed in either group.

Table 7 Objective side-effects. Occurrence in individual cycles

| | | | | Cycle | | | |
	P	1	2	3	4	5	6
Femodene							
Acne	5 (3%)	7 (4%)	6 (3%)	5 (3%)	6 (3%)	4 (2%)	6 (4%)
Chloasma	—	—	—	1 (1%)	—	—	
Edema	1 (1%)	—	—	—	1 (1%)	—	–
Microgynon 30							
Acne	3 (2%)	2 (1%)	3 (2%)	5 (3%)	3 (2%)	2 (1%)	4 (3%)
Chloasma	—	—	—	1 (1%)	1 (1%)	—	1 (1%)
Edema	1 (1%)	2 (1%)	1 (1%)	3 (2%)	—	—	1 (1%)

P = Last pretreatment cycle.
No cases of thrombophlebitis or liver disease were reported.

Of the subjective side-effects (Figure 8) the most common in both groups were headaches, depression, nausea and breast tension. Compare Tables 11 and 12 for the pretreatment level of complaints. All other side-effects were relatively infrequent. The incidence of headaches and depression was similar in the 2 treatment groups and in both cases was higher in the 1st 3 cycles. Nausea was common in the Microgynon group, but again mainly in the 1st 3 cycles. Breast tension was more frequent and affected more patients (14%) in the Femodene

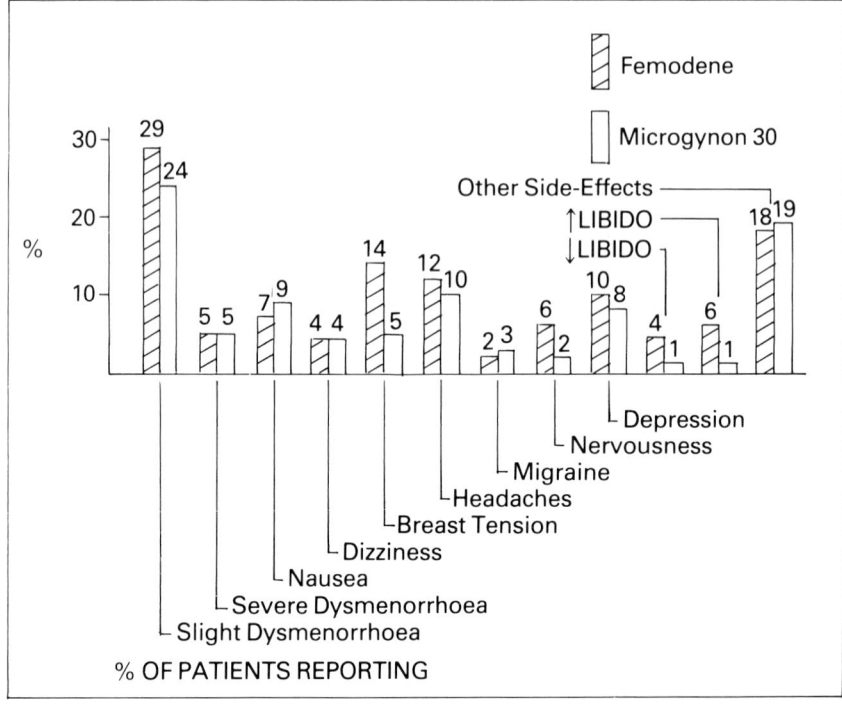

Figure 8   Subjective side-effects, cycles 1–6

group, again mainly in the 1st 3 cycles. The incidence of other side-effects, not categorized on the case report form, was similar in both groups and was fairly constant throughout the study.

PHASE III – OPEN ASSESSMENT OF FEMODENE

Included in this assessment are the 189 patients originally recruited to the Femodene group in the study, plus 122 patients who were switched from Microgynon to Femodene after 6 cycles. Admission data on these latter were updated on entry to the open assessment phase. Of the total group, therefore, 74% of patients had used a combined oral contraceptive during the 3 months prior to entry.

Data are available from only 60 patients for the full 18 cycles, but 3067 cycles have so far been analyzed (Figure 9). Withdrawals to date are shown in Table 8. Only 17 patients (5%) have been lost to follow-up so far.

Three patients have been withdrawn due to pregnancy (Table 9).

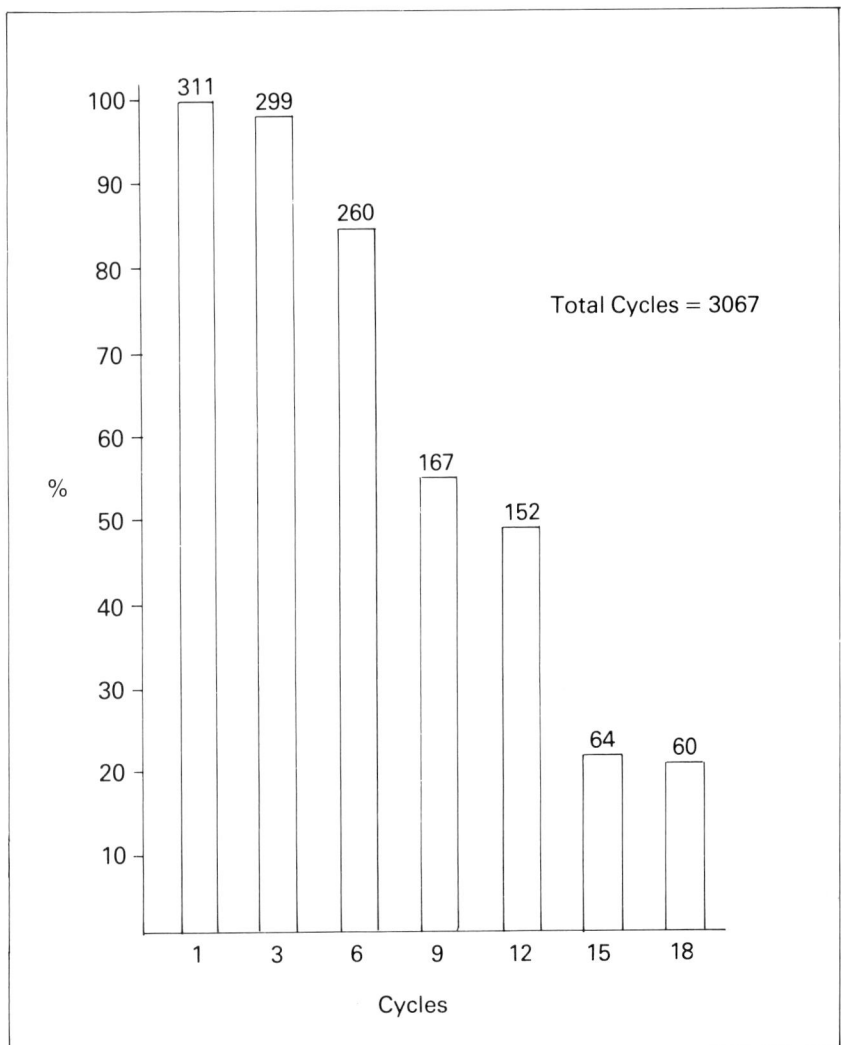

Figure 9   Recruitment and number of patients completing cycles

In 2 out of 3 cases errors in tablet taking have been assumed to be the reason for contraceptive failure.

Only 10% of the total cycles showed intermenstrual bleeding, and of those cycles where single tablets were known to have been missed still 80% were free of any intermenstrual bleeding (Table 10).

Changes in body weight are shown in Figure 10.

Table 8 Patients withdrawn from or failing to complete the study

| | | Number (and percentage of totals) of patients | | | | |
| | | Reason for withdrawal or drop-out | | | | |
	Side-effects	Pregnant	Lost to follow up	Contra-ception not wanted	Other reasons	Total
Cycle 1	7	—	1	—	—	8 (3%)
2	3	—	—	1	—	4 (1%)
3	8	—	5	2	5	20 (6%)
4–6	12	2	8	4	8	34 (11%)
7–12	13	—	3	3	9	28 (9%)
13–18	1	1	—	2	2	6 (2%)
All cycles	44	3	17	12	24	100
	(14%)	(1%)	(5%)	(4%)	(12%)	(32%)

Table 9 Pregnancies occurring during the study

Patient 286	Pregnancy detected following 6th cycle of Femodene
	Diagnosed as 3 months pregnant at that time
	Had missed 2 tablets in cycle 3,
	1 tablet in cycle 4,
	1 tablet in cycle 5,
	and 1 tablet in cycle 6
Patient 471	Pregnancy detected following 16th cycle of Femodene
	Diagnosed as 1 month pregnant at that time
	No missed tablets had been recorded
Patient 477	Pregnancy detected following 6th cycle of Femodene
	Diagnosed as 2 months pregnant at that time
	Had missed 1 tablet in cycle 4,
	5 tablets in cycle 5,
	and 5 tablets in cycle 6

Table 10 Intermenstrual bleeding during complete and incomplete tablet taking

Cycles with no missed tablets:
Cycles 1–18   intermenstrual bleeding = 9%
                                              breakthrough bleeding = 4%

Cycles with tablets missed:
Cycles 1–18   intermenstrual bleeding = 20%
                                              breakthrough bleeding = 10%

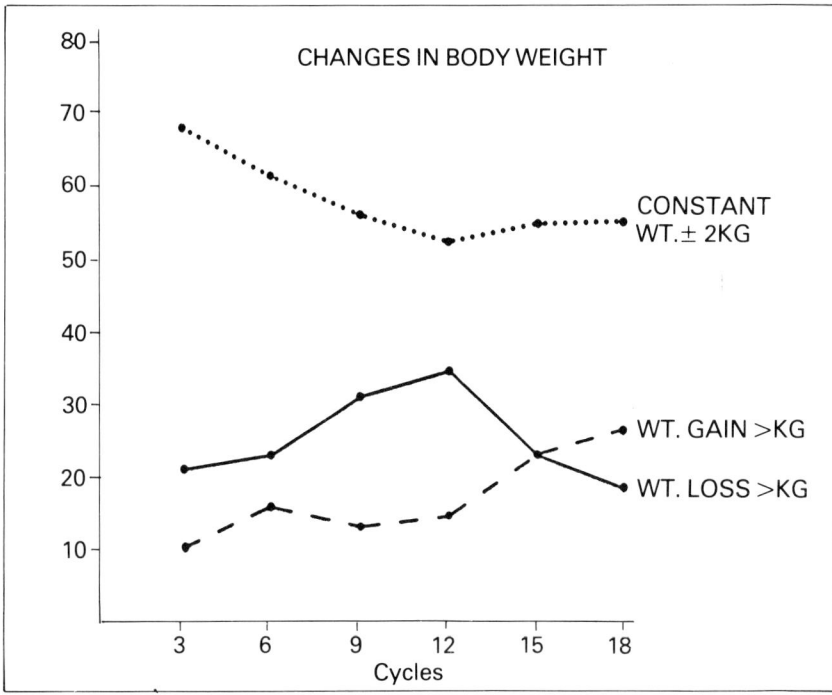

Figure 10 Changes in body weight

Of the objective side-effects (Table 11) acne was the most frequently reported, but occurred during the 1st 6 cycles at a rate (3%) unchanged from the pretreatment cycle. Numbers involved are too small to assess in later cycles.

Of the subjective side-effects (Table 12) breast tension was reported at some time by 14% of patients at a rate highest during the 1st 3 cycles (6% of patients during each of those cycles compared to 1% of patients during the pretreatment cycle). Headaches were the next most frequently reported, but with an incidence of 5% in each of the 1st 3 cycles – not much different from the pretreatment cycle incidence.

Table 11 Number of patients reporting objective side-effects

	P	*In cycles 1 to 3*	*In cycles 4 to 6*	*In cycles 7 to 12*	*In cycles 13 to 18*	*Overall*
Acne	9 (3%)	12 (4%)	15 (5%)	8 (5%)	3 (5%)	25 (8%)
Chloasma	1 (1%)	2 (1%)	—	—	—	2 (1%)
Edema	1 (1%)	2 (1%)	2 (1%)	—	—	3 (1%)

P = pretreatment cycle.
No cases of thrombophlebitis or liver disease were reported.

Table 12 Subjective side-effects – occurrence in individual cycles (percentage)

			Cycle			
	P	*1*	*3*	*6*	*12*	*18*
Dysmenorrhea:						
Slight	19	9	11	15	12	12
Severe	5	1	2	1	1	—
Nausea	4	3	1	2	1	—
Vomiting	—	1	2	1	—	—
Dizziness	—	1	1	1	1	—
Breast tension	1	6	6	4	4	—
Varicose complaints	1	1	1	—	—	—
Headaches	4	5	5	3	3	3
Migraine	—	1	1	1	1	—
Nervousness	1	2	1	1	—	—
Depression	2	3	5	3	3	—
↑libido	—	—	1	1	—	—
↓libido	1	1	2	1	1	—
Others	5	7	7	9	4	3

Likewise, nausea, whilst reported by 21 patients overall, still had only a 1% higher incidence in the 1st cycle than in the pretreatment cycle.

Forty-four patients (14%) have withdrawn due to side-effects, mostly multiple, but including mood changes (irritability or depression) in 15 patients, abnormal bleeding in 13 patients, unacceptable weight gain in 9 patients and migrainous headaches in 5 patients (Table 13).

Table 13 Withdrawals due to side-effects

Complaints were mainly multiple, the most common were:

Number of patients	*Side-effect*
15	Irritability or depression
13	Abnormal bleeding
9	Unacceptable weight gain
5	Migrainous headaches
5	Breast tension

These findings support in general those of the European Study. No severe side-effects have occurred throughout the period of treatment. The new pill gives better cycle control than Microgynon 30, with lower progestogen dosage and whilst retaining the simplicity of a monophasic formulation.

Femodene has been very well tolerated by our patients, particularly since there is a tendency to over-report side-effects when patients know they are taking part in a trial.

9

A study of the metabolic effects of monophasic gestodene and desogestrel preparations

P. G. Crosignani, F. Vergadoro, G. A. Giudici, G. Vigotti,
C. Vergani, F. Franceschetti, B. Cesana and R. Orlandi

Lowering the estrogen dose of oral contraceptives did not substantially decrease the frequency of arterial thromboembolic disease[1] and this is probably linked to the tendency to lower the HDL-cholesterol fraction induced by the effect of the progestogen present in the pills[2]. HDL-cholesterol, which is considered to have a protective vascular effect[3] is favourably increased by estrogen[4]. The undesirable progestogenic effect on lipoprotein is generally ascribed to the residual intrinsic androgenic activity of the 19-norderivative component of the oral contraceptive[5].

A recent preparation containing desogestrel seems to show a more favourable effect on the lipoprotein pattern and in particular does not interfere with the estrogen-induced rise in HDL-cholesterol[2-6].

More recently the new 19-norderivative – gestodene – has been made available. In the preclinical and first clinical studies this compound showed negligible effects on lipid metabolism.

The purpose of our randomized single-blind study was to compare metabolic parameters for matched healthy female volunteers taking 2 different oral contraceptives: Preparation A – Femodene – (30 μg ethinyl estradiol + 75 μg gestodene) and Preparation B – Marvelon – (30 μg ethinyl estradiol + 150 μg desogestrel), both containing new progestogens.

PATIENTS AND METHODS

Tablets containing Preparation A were administered orally to 10 healthy volunteers and Preparation B to 12. Their mean age was 21.5 years (S.D. 3.02 – range 18–30).

Exclusion criteria were:

(1) women with contra-indications to oral contraceptives; or
(2) puerperal women (fewer than 3 cycles after delivery/lactation);
(3) women on drugs (long-term treatment with drugs that act on lipids and drugs interacting with oral contraceptives);
(4) women who smoked more than 10 cigarettes per day;
(5) women who were on dietary regimes.

The women were instructed to take the first pill on the 1st day of the cycle and for 21 consecutive days and to start the treatment again after a medication-free interval of 7 days.

Fasting morning blood samples were drawn during the luteal phase of the pretreatment cycle (days 21–24) and after 3 and 6 months of therapy. Total cholesterol, triglycerides, phospholipids, VLDL-cholesterol, LDL-cholesterol, HDL-cholesterol, HDL_2-cholesterol, HDL_3-cholesterol and glucose were determined within 4 hours after venesection, while sex-hormone-binding globulin (SHBG), free testosterone, Apoliprotein A_1 (Apo A_1), Apoliprotein B (Apo B) and immunoreactive insulin were kept frozen until assayed. Blood was taken at cycles 0, 3, and 6, whereas oral glucose tolerance tests (OGTT) and immunoreactive insulin tests were performed at cycles 0 and 6. Total cholesterol, triglycerides, phospholipids and glucose were determined by enzymatic methods (Boehringer, Mannheim, FRG). The HDL-cholesterol was determined by the two-step precipitation method of Gidez et al.[7] The OGTT was performed as described by the National Diabetes Data Group[8] Apo A_1 and Apo B were determined by single radial immuno-diffusion (RID), using standards provided by the manufacturer. SHBG was measured as binding capacity toward DHT-3H. The SHBG-DHT complex was separated by ammonium sulphate precipitation, while radio-immunoassay of free testosterone was carried out using the coated tubes DPC method. The data were evaluated statistically by multifactoral mixed Ancova.

RESULTS AND DISCUSSION

Table 1 shows the mean data for the single parameters before and during the treatment.

There were no changes in total cholesterol, LDL-cholesterol, Apo B or phospholipids levels from basal levels in either group. HDL-cholesterol levels increased during the treatment in both groups, but the rise was significant only for women taking Preparation A.

No 'between groups' differences were observed at any time. Several

Table 1   Plasma concentrations before and during the treatments (absolute values and Δ %).

			Basal		After 3 months			After 6 months		
		N.	X̄	d.s.	X̄	d.s.	Δ%	X̄	d.s.	Δ%
Total cholesterol										
Femodene	0	9	165	28.1	177	22.5	+ 7.6	177	37.1	+ 7.1
Marvelon	00	12	176	40.7	173	31.2	− 1.6	183	41.8	+ 4.0
Triglycerides	0	9	78	38.7	96.7	29.0	+ 23.4	100.7	33.1	+ 28.5
	00	12	65	18.9	90.6*	29.9	+ 39.4	99.6*	30.6	+ 53.2
VLDL	0	8	11.9	3.3	21.8	13.26	+ 83.2	21.8	9.22	+ 83.2
	00	12	12.9	3.7	18.0*	5.95	+ 39.4	20.0*	6.13	+ 54.8
LDL	0	8	98.9	27.5	95.6	23.75	− 3.3	94.5	26.45	− 4.4
	00	12	108.4	36.0	94.1	35.42	− 13.2	107.3	40.94	− 1.1
HDL	0	10	53.3	9.5	57.5*	8.22	+ 7.9	61.4*	9.65	+ 15.2
	00	12	53.7	12.3	61.0	11.44	+ 13.7	55.6	11.74	+ 3.6
HDL$_2$	0	10	24.3	9.2	20.2	10.94	− 16.9	24.3	6.34	− 0.0
	00	10	25.5	13.6	25.4	9.47	+ 0.8	20.6	12.94	− 19.2
HDL$_3$	0	11	29.0	3.3	35.7	6.86	+ 23.1	36.1	7.09	+ 24.5
	00	10	28.2	8.2	35.1*	4.87	+ 24.5	35.4*	5.66	+ 25.5
APO A	0	11	136	25.4	145*	23.7	+ 7.0	160*	18.5	+ 18.2
	00	8	133	23.1	148*	23.7	+ 11.7	150*	31.4	+ 13.1
APO B	0	11	81	23.1	81	19.9	− 0.6	90	20.2	+ 11.2
	00	8	77	11.1	83	12.9	+ 8.9	92	24.4	+ 19.8
Oral glucose tolerance	0	11	80	6.8	—	—		85	4.8	+ 6.3
	00	10	79	7.7	—	—		82	6.8	+ 4.0
Phospholipids	0	12	172	22.1	170	59.7	− 0.87	210	35.6	+ 22.2
	00	8	179	30.4	208	79.5	+ 16.3	201	38.1	+ 12.8
SHGB	0	11	22.4	5.2	50.1*	3.26	+ 123.5	50.9*	4.99	+ 126.8
	00	7	17.9	4.2	43.9*	11.83	+ 145.7	45.3*	12.33	+ 153.3
Free testosterone	0	8	2.60	0.97	0.83*	0.455	− 68.0	0.82*	0.477	− 68.0
	00	7	2.99	0.98	1.03*	0.377	− 65.6	1.01*	0.416	− 66.3

p between times * *p* < 0.01
p between drugs = n.s.
Multifactoral mixed Ancova test (drug and time: fixed factors at 2 levels patient random factor nested in the drug factor with repeated measurements for the same subject. The basal value was taken as the covariate)

HDL-cholesterol studies have been done in women taking Preparation B, some indicating significant rises[6,9,10], others no change[11,12].

The HDL_2-cholesterol subfraction (the subfraction which apparently protects against atherosclerosis) did not change in either group and therefore the rise in HDL probably reflects an increse in HDL_3[13].

Apo A_1 is significantly increased in both groups, this effect probably being due to the estrogenic component of the pill[4].

Table 1 shows the trends of changes in lipoprotein ($\Delta\%$). The effect of sex hormones on serum lipoproteins has been extensively studied, but the underlying mechanisms are still poorly understood. Estrogens may affect lipoprotein metabolism in different ways. They decrease hepatic triglyceride lipase activity[13,14], which can lead to an increase in HDL. Estrogen also enhances the hepatic synthesis of VLDL, Apo B and Apo A[15,16]. Progestogen 19-norderivatives, because of their residual intrinsic androgenic activity, can increase both hepatic and extrahepatic lipase activities[17,18], possibly decreasing HDL and triglyceride concentrations.

Progestogens, 17-OH derivatives with low or absent androgenic activity (MPA and CPA), have been reported to have no effect on lipoprotein concentrations[19,20].

The unchanged total cholesterol values and the preferential distribution of cholesterol into the HDL fraction might be related to an increase of Apo A_1 directing cholesterol to the non-atherogenic HDL fraction.

The oral glucose tolerance test showed no significant increase (6.3% with Femodene and 4% with Marvelon) in hyperglycemia at 6 months in both groups. No one individual response was above the limits of normal. Basal immunoreactive insulin did not change during either treatment but the data are limited (6 and 7 subjects for the 2 groups respectively) and are for the 3-month samples only.

As expected, SHBG was significantly increased by both treatments, and as a consequence there was a significant reduction in free testosterone. There were no differences between groups in SHBG or free testosterone at any time.

In conclusion, the data obtained and the lack of significant differences between drugs at all times indicate that the two pills have equal, very low and, theoretically, no adverse metabolic effects.

REFERENCES

1. Bottiger, L.E., Boman, G., Eklund, G. and Westerholm, B. (1980). Oral contraceptives and thromboembolic disease: effects of lowering oestrogen content. *Lancet*, i, 1097–101.

2. Wynn, V. and Nithyanthan, R. (1982). The effect of progestins in combined oral contraceptives on serum lipids with special references to high-density lipoproteins. *Am. J. Obstet. Gynecol.*, **142**, 766–72.
3. Miller, G. J. and Miller, N. E. (1975). Plasma high density lipoprotein concentration and development of ischaemic heart disease. *Lancet*, **i**, 16–19.
4. Patsch, W., Kim, K., Wiest, W. and Schonfeld, G. (1980). Effects of sex hormones on rat lipoproteins. *Endocrinology*, **107**, 1085–94.
5. Knopp, R. H., Walden, C. E., Wahl, P. W. and Hoover, J. J. (1982). Effects of oral contraceptives on lipoprotein triglyceride and cholesterol: relationships to estrogen and progestin potency. *Am. J. Obstet. Gynecol.*, **142**, 725–31.
6. Samsioe, G. (1982). Comparative effects of the oral contraceptive combinations 0.150 mg desogestrel + 0.030 mg ethinyl-oestradiol and 0.150 mg levonorgestrel + 0.030 mg ethinyl-oestradiol on lipids and lipoprotein metabolism in healthy female volunteers. *Contraception*, **25**, 487–504.
7. Gidez, L. I., Miller, G. J., Burstein, M. *et al.* (1982). Separation and quantitation of subclasses of human density lipoprotein subclasses by a single precipitation procedure. *J. Lipid. Res.*, **23**, 1206.
8. National Diabetes Data Group (1979). Classification and diagnosis of diabetes mellitus and other categories of glucose intolerance. *Diabetes*, **29**, 1039.
9. Wiseman, A., Bowie, J. and Cogswell, D. (1984). Marvelon: Clinical experience in the U. K. *Br. J. Fam. Plan.*, **10**, 38–42.
10. Bergink, E. W., Borglin, N. E., Klottrup, P. and Linklo, P. (1982). Effects of desogestrel in low dose oestrogen oral contraceptives on serum lipoproteins. *Contraception*, **25**, 477–85.
11. Cullberg, G., Samsioe, G., Andersen, R. F., Bredesgaard, P., Andersen, N. B., Ernerot, H., Fanoe, E., Fylling, P., Haack-Soresen, P. E., Klottrup, P., Pedersen, J. H. and Sandager, T. (1982). Two oral contraceptives, efficacy, serum proteins and lipid metabolism: a comparative multicenter study on a triphasic and fixed dose combination. *Contraception*, **26**, 229–42.
12. Godsland, I. F. and Wynn, V. (1984). Does the new progestogen desogestrel have metabolic advantages? *Lancet*, **ii**, 359–60.
13. Glueck, C. T., Fallat, R. W. and Scheel, D. (1975). Effects of estrogenic compounds on triglyceride kinetics. *Metabolism*, **24**, 537.
14. Appelbaum, D., Goldeberg, A. P. and Pykalisto, O. J. (1977). Effect of estrogen on post heparin lipolitic activity. Selective decline in hepatic triglyceride lipase. *J. Clin. Invest.*, **59**, 601.
15. Jansen, H., Vantol, A. and Hulsmann, W. C. (1980). On the metabolic function of heparin releasable liver lipase. *Biochem. Biophys. Res. Comm.*, **92**, 53.
16. Kunsi, T., Saarinen, P. and Nikkila, E. A. (1980). Evidence for the mode of hepatic endothelial lipase in metabolism of high density lipoproteins in man. *Atherosclerosis*, **361**, 589.
17. Schalfer, E. J., Zech, L. A., Jenkins, L. L., Bronzert, J. J., Rubalcaba, E. A., Lindgren, F. T., Aamodt, R. L. and Brewer Jr, H. B. (1982). Human apoliprotein AI and AII metabolism. *J. Lipid. Res.*, **57**, 850.
18. Schalfer, E. T., Fostec, D. M., Zech, L. A., Lindgren, F. T., Brewer Jr, H. B. and Levy, R. J. (1983). The effect of estrogen administration on plasma lipoprotein metabolism in premenopausal women. *J. Clin. Metab. Endocrinol.*, **57**, 262.
19. Glueck, C. J., Gartside, P., Fallat, R. W. and Mendoza, S. (1976). Effect of sex hormones on protamine mactivated and resistant post heparin plasma lipases. *Metabolism*, **25**, 625.
20. Tikkanen, M., Nikkila, E. A., Kuusi, T. and Sipinen, S. (1981). Reduction of plasma high-density lipoprotein, cholesterol and increase of post herapin plasma hepatic lipase activity during progestogen treatment. *Clin. Chim. Acta*, **115**, 63.

21. Hirvonen, E., Mälkönen, M. and Manninen, V. (1981). Effects of different pro-
    gestogens on lipoproteins during postmenopausal replacement therapy. *N. Engl.
    J. Med.*, **304**, 560.

22. Tikkanen, M., Nikkila, E. A., Kuusi, T. and Sipinen, S. (1981). Different effects of
    two progestins on plasma high density lipoprotein (HDL_2) and post heparin
    plasma hepatic lipase activity. *Atherosclerosis*, **40**, 365.

10

Metabolic effects of Femodene in new users, long-term users, and users switched from other oral contraceptives: an interim analysis

P. Bye

INTRODUCTION

Since the clinical detection of rare side-effects, and the comparison of their incidences with different pills, are inevitably lengthy processes, clues are sought for any potential adverse effects in the metabolic changes, often of a very minor degree, that pills produce.

MATERIAL AND METHODS

Three groups of women taking gestodene (GES) 75 μg + ethinyl estradiol 30 μg (Femodene) daily for 21 days in each 28 days are being studied.*

New users: 14 healthy women aged 17–33 (22.8 ± 1.7 SEM)**, who had used no hormonal contraception in the previous 6 months and who had had at least 3 regular cycles post partum or post abortum.

Switch users: 13 healthy women aged 20–34 (27.7 ± 1.3 SEM) who had taken other low-estrogen oral contraceptives (in one case a progestogen-only pill) for at least the last 6 cycles.

Long-term users: 15 healthy women aged 17–33 (25.1 ± 1.2 SEM) who had taken Femodene for 11–18 cycles (15.4 ± 0.6 SEM).

Exclusion criteria: weight > 25% above or below ideal; sitting diastolic pressure > 90 mm Hg; existing or latent diabetes; pathological hyperlipidemia; taking drugs that affect plasma lipids, or any regular medication; taking a reducing (or varying) diet; smoking > 10 cigarettes/day.

Sampling: Fasting blood samples were taken on one day per cycle

---

* The clinical study was supervised by Dr Bernadette Lee and the laboratory analysis by Dr Ken Fotherby.
** SEM = standard error of the mean.

(days 14–21). New users were sampled in the last pretreatment cycle and in treatment cycles 1, 3, and 6. Switch users were sampled in each of the last two pretreatment cycles and in each of cycles 1–6 on Femodene. Long-term users were sampled once.

Parameters studied: Factor X, antithrombin III, total cholesterol, fractionated lipoprotein cholesterol, total triglycerides, glucose and insulin (oral glucose tolerance test), sex-hormone-binding globulin (SHBG), caeruloplasmin, gamma-glutamyl transferase.

Analysis: The mean values are presented as percentages of the untreated means (new users) or of the mean values while taking the previous pills (switch users). The data from the long-term users are related to the latest values in the other groups by linking them with broken lines. Normal laboratory ranges are indicated, except in the figures that include HDL fractions.

RESULTS

Coagulation system: In new users, only Femodene showed any indication of a fall in factor X (Figure 1). The impression seems to be confirmed in switch users, in all of whom factor X fell, the mean reaching the lower limit of normal (Figure 2).

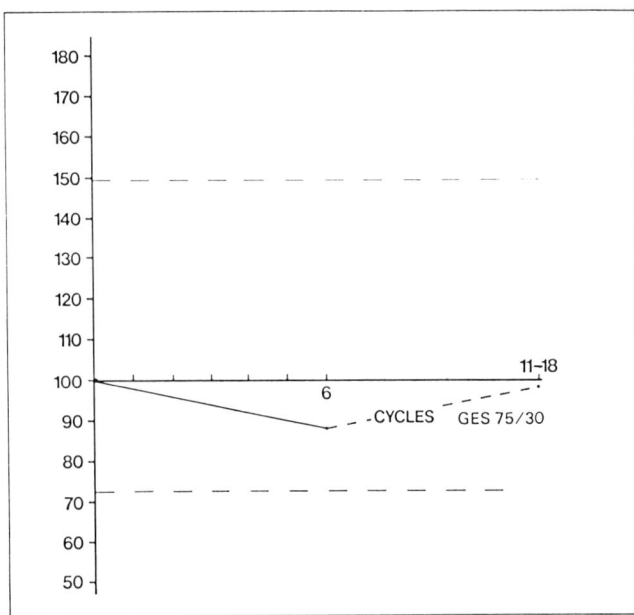

Figure 1   Factor X – new users

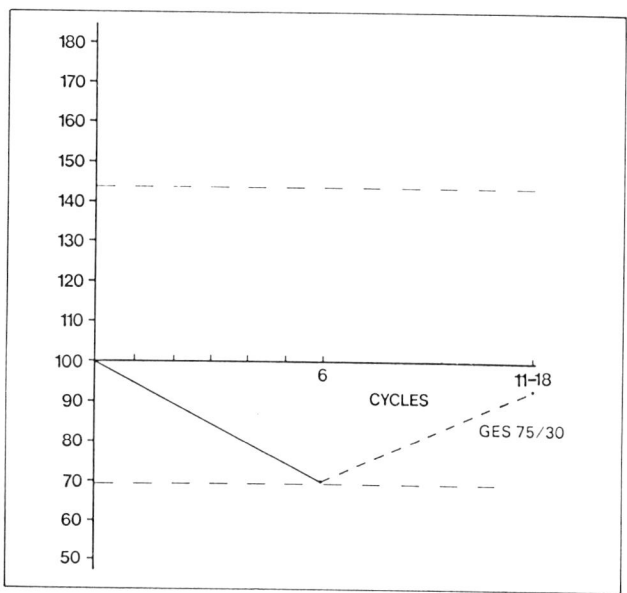

Figure 2   Factor X – switch users

Mean antithrombin III fell slightly in new users of all the pills (Figure 3). Eight out of 10 long-term users of other pills were below the normal range, but on switching to Femodene 7 out of 9 rose into the normal range (Figure 4).

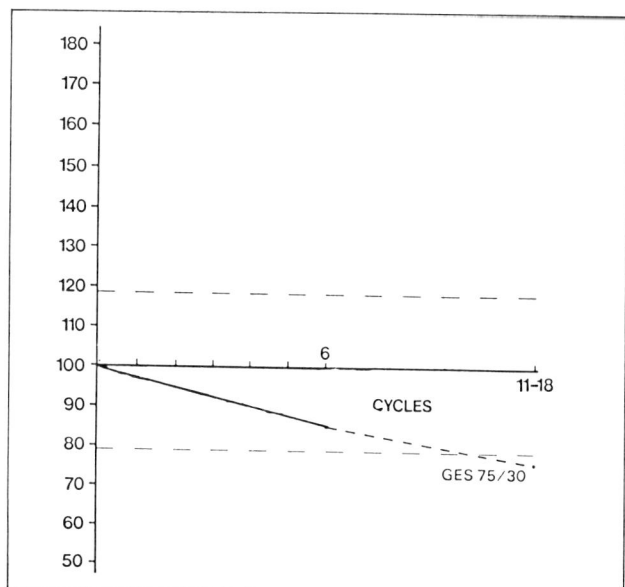

Figure 3   Antithrombin III – new users

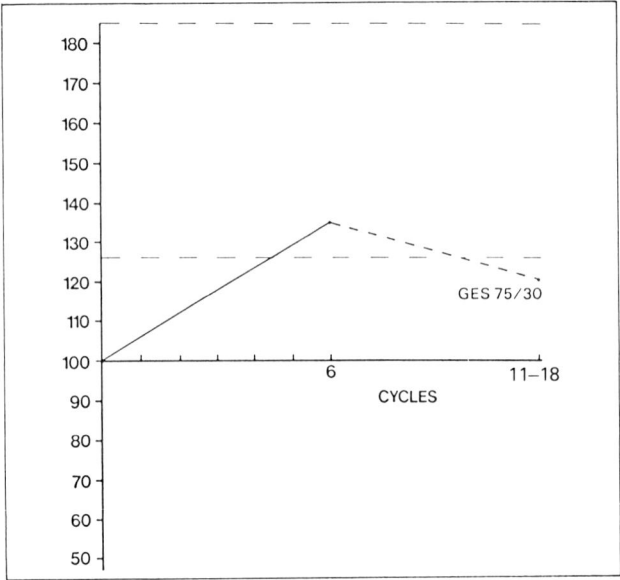

Figure 4   Antithrombin III – switch users

Plasma lipids: Total cholesterol rose hardly at all in new users, as with the other low-estrogen pills (Figure 5) and also showed no difference between previous pills and Femodene in switch users (Figure 6).

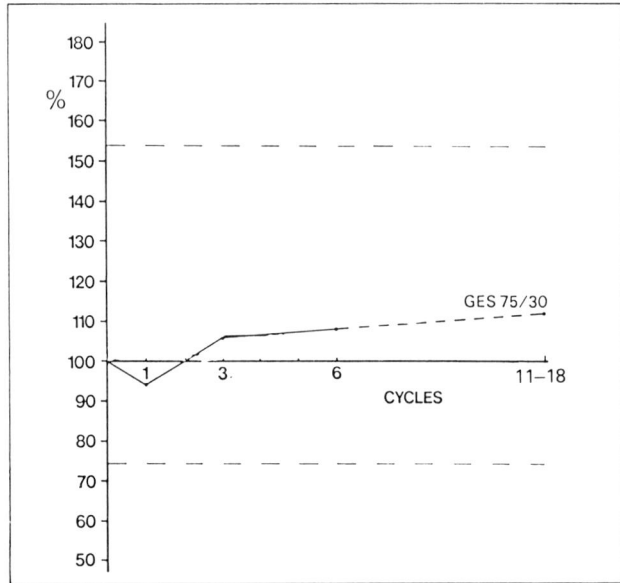

Figure 5   Total cholesterol – new users

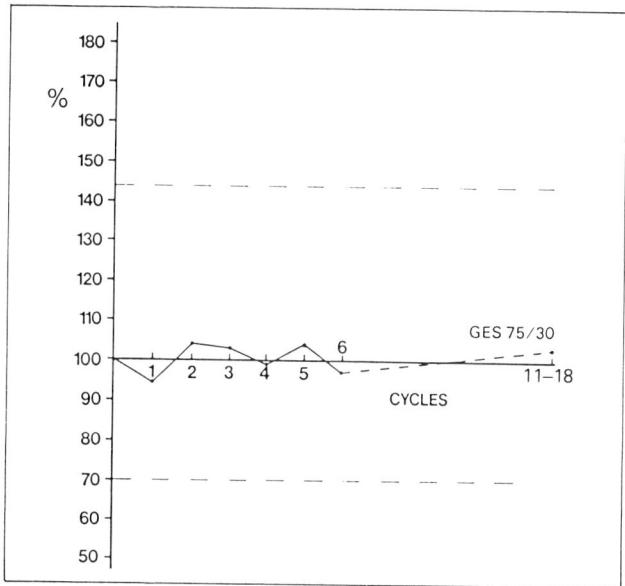

Figure 6 Total cholesterol – switch users

Triglycerides (TG) rose significantly, and more with Femodene than with the other pills, both in new users (Figure 7) and initially in switch users (Figure 8), but the level in long-term users was no higher than in the users of other pills before the switch. There was a significant

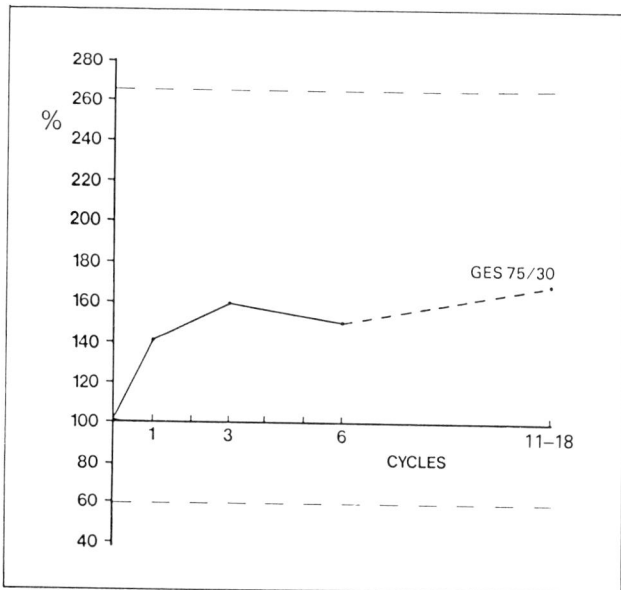

Figure 7 Triglycerides – new users

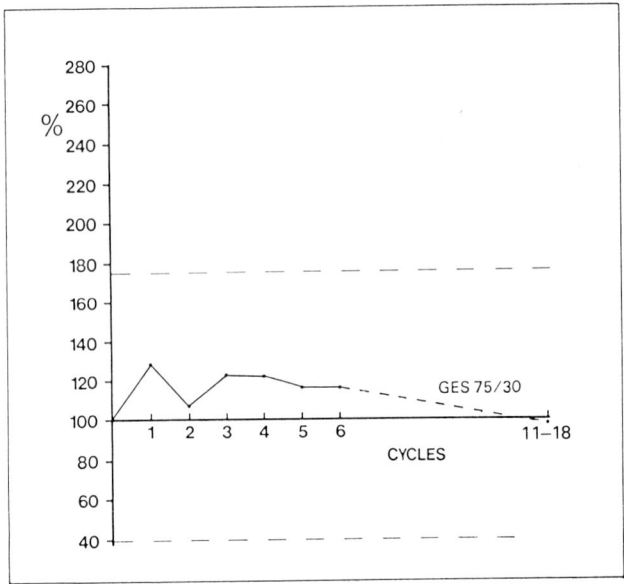

Figure 8   Triglycerides – switch users

rise in very-low-density lipoproteins (VLDL) comparable with the rise
in TG in new users (Figure 9), and a small but sustained rise in switch
users (Figure 10). Low-density lipoproteins (LDL) showed no change
within 6 months in new users (Figure 11) and the switch users show

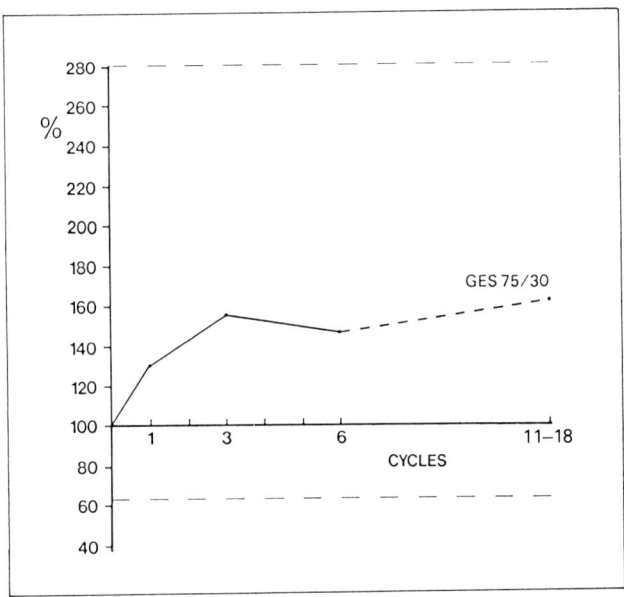

Figure 9   VLDL-cholesterol – new users

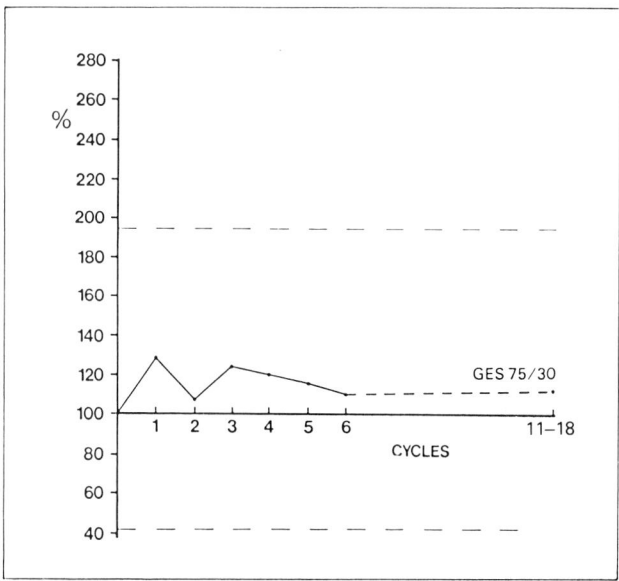

Figure 10   VLDL-cholesterol – switch users

that the higher LDL seen in long-term users is no higher than the level existing in long-term users of the other pills (Figure 12).

HDL$_2$ fell initially in new users, but was higher at 6 months (Figure 13). In the switch users, HDL$_2$ fluctuated above and below the previous

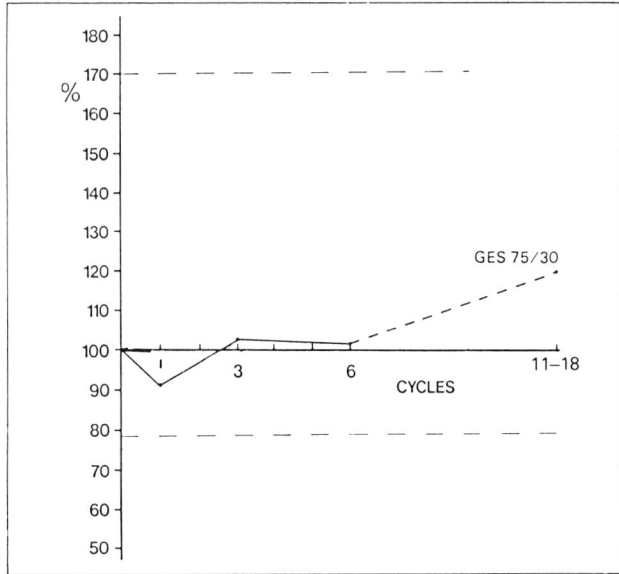

Figure 11   LDL-cholesterol – new users

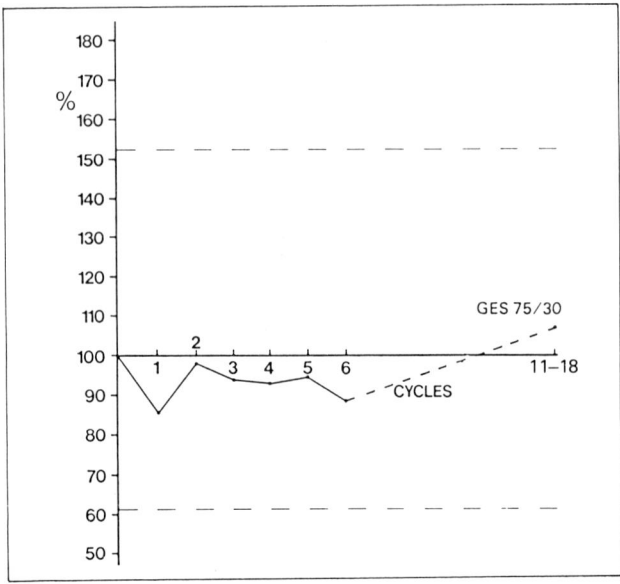

Figure 12   LDL-cholesterol – switch users

level (Figure 14). HDL$_3$ showed a rise at 6 months in new users (Figure 15) and a marked increase from the 2nd cycle onwards in the switch users, though not in the long-term users (Figure 16).

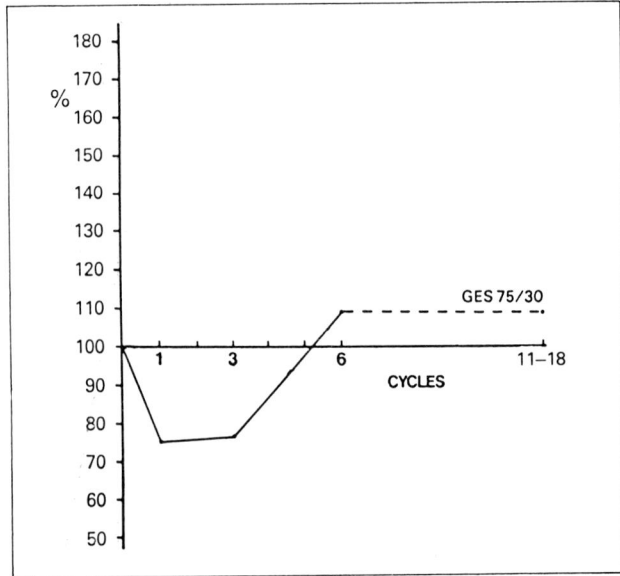

Figure 13   HDL$_2$ – new users

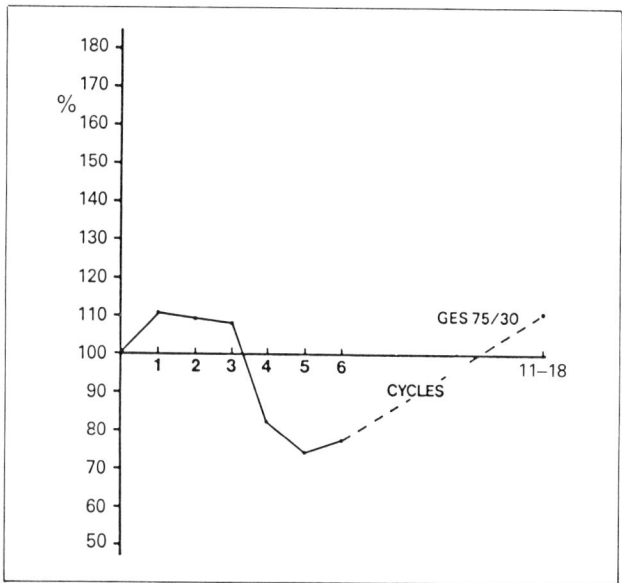

Figure 14   HDL$_2$ – switch users

The ratios of HDL to total cholesterol (Figure 17) and HDL to non-HDL-cholesterol* (Figure 18) rose on switching to Femodene, while

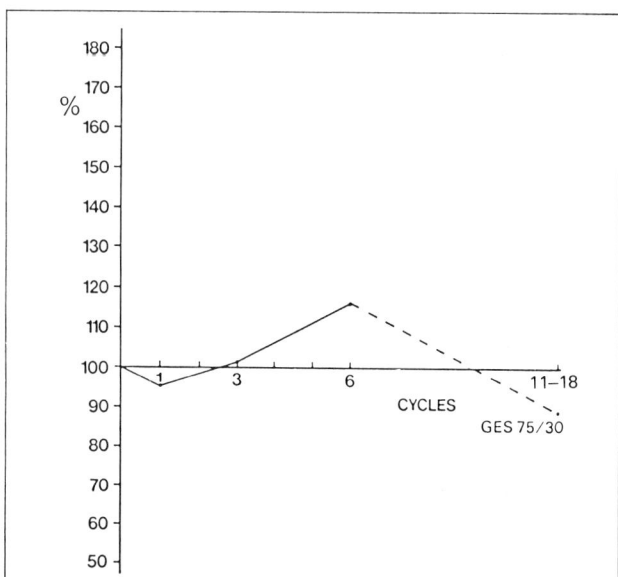

Figure 15   HDL$_3$ – new users

* Non-HDL-cholesterol = total lipoprotein-cholesterol minus HDL-cholesterol.

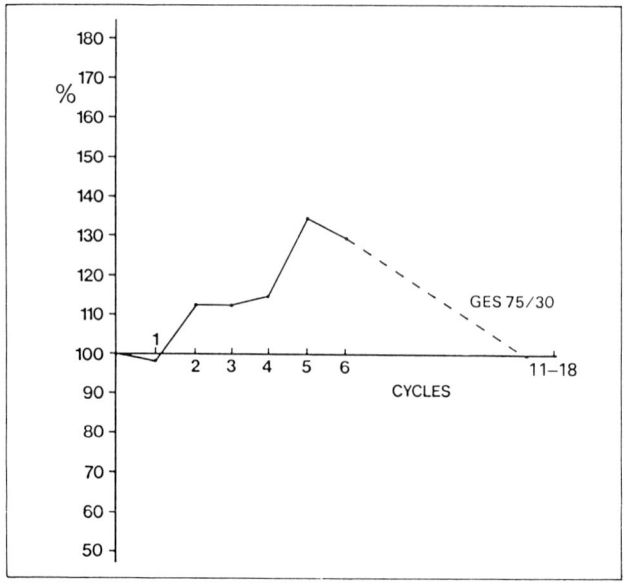

Figure 16   HDL₃ – switch users

the ratio of HDL$_2$ to LDL (Figure 19) showed a marked rise in the 1st cycle after switching but thereafter fluctuated around the original level. Figure 20 shows 3 HDL ratios. Small but insignificant rises in

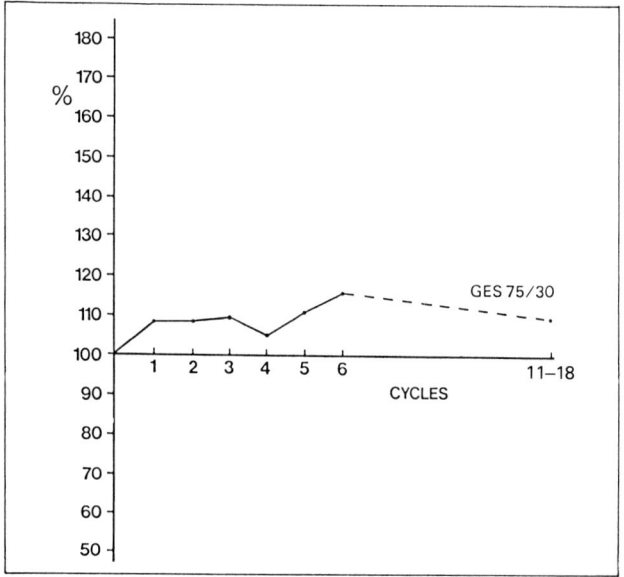

Figure 17   HDL-cholesterol: total cholesterol – switch users

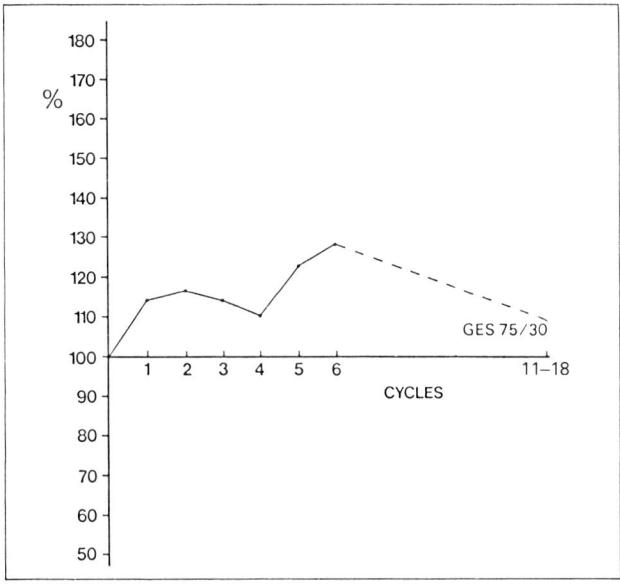

Figure 18   HDL:non-HDL-cholesterol – switch users

all ratios occurred with Femodene.

Glucose tolerance tests ($n = 6$) showed a moderate rise in glucose

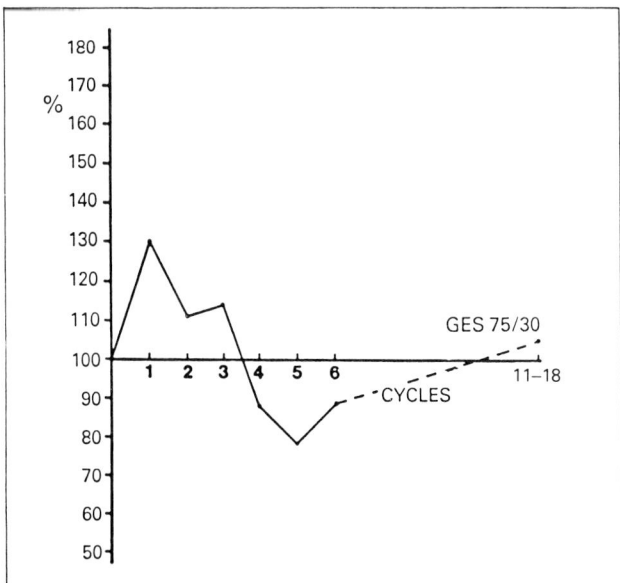

Figure 19   HDL$_2$:LDL-cholesterol – switch users

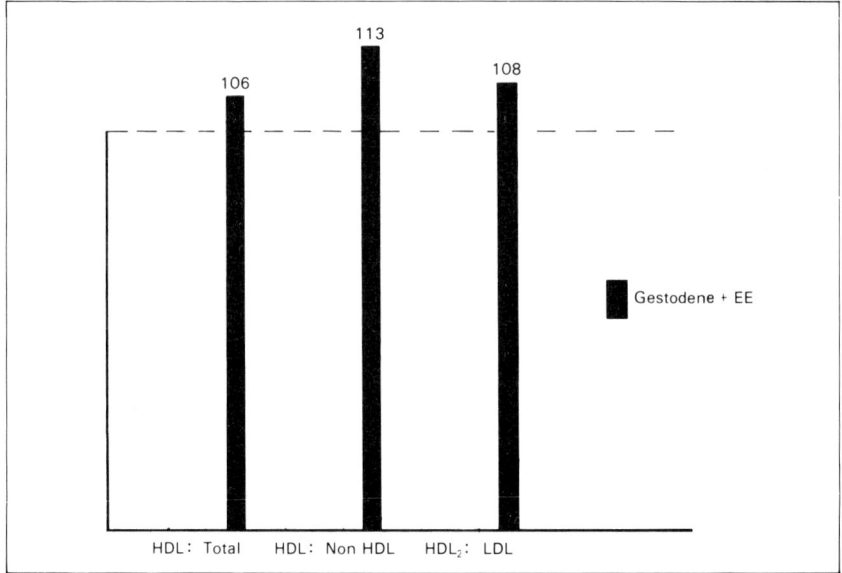

Figure 20   Ratios of lipoprotein fractions at 6th cycle as percentages of pre-treatment ratios

levels, but the mean insulin level was not increased by Femodene (Figures 21 and 22).

Serum gamma-glutamyl transferase (an index of liver function) rose in new users, and showed a rise after 6 cycles in switch users, but was similar to initial levels in long-term users (Figures 23 and 24). The

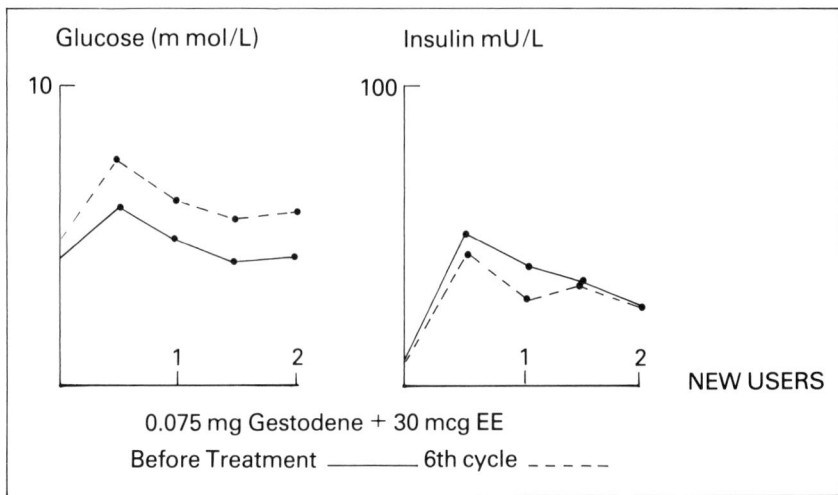

Figure 21   Glucose tolerance tests – new users

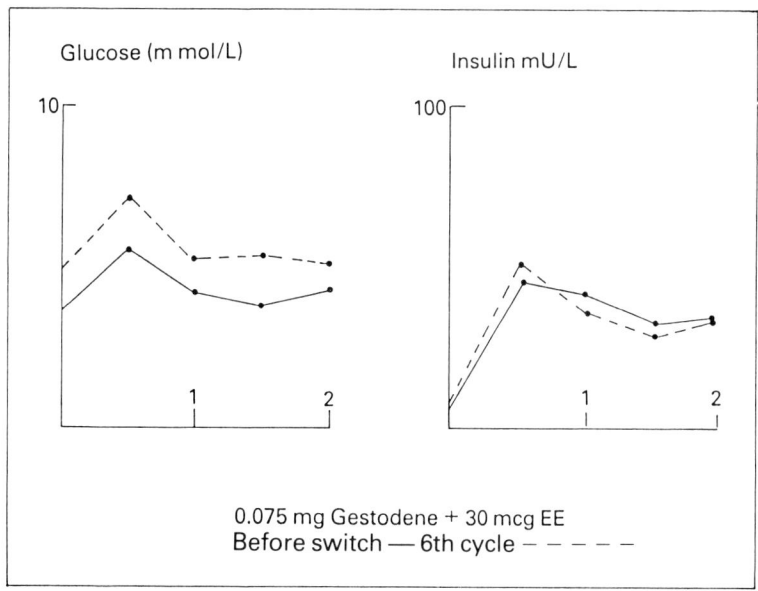

Figure 22   Glucose tolerance tests – switch users

estrogen-sensitive protein, caeruloplasmin, rose markedly in new users (Figure 25), but not in switch users (Figure 26), whereas SHBG rose in both (Figures 27 and 28).

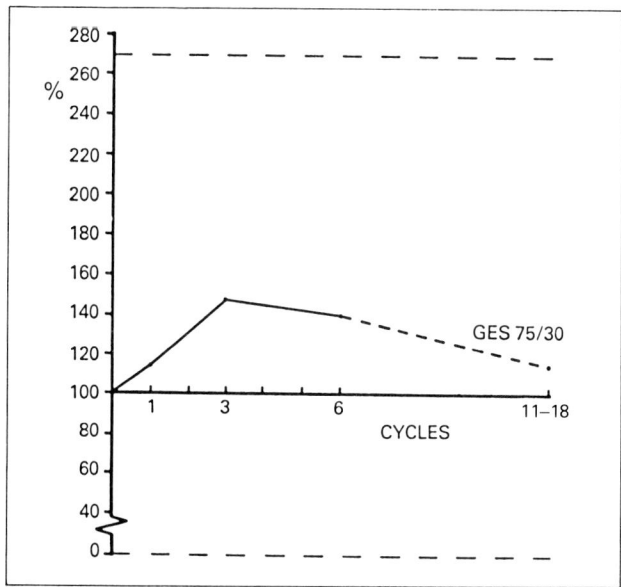

Figure 23   Serum gamma-glutamyl transferase – new users

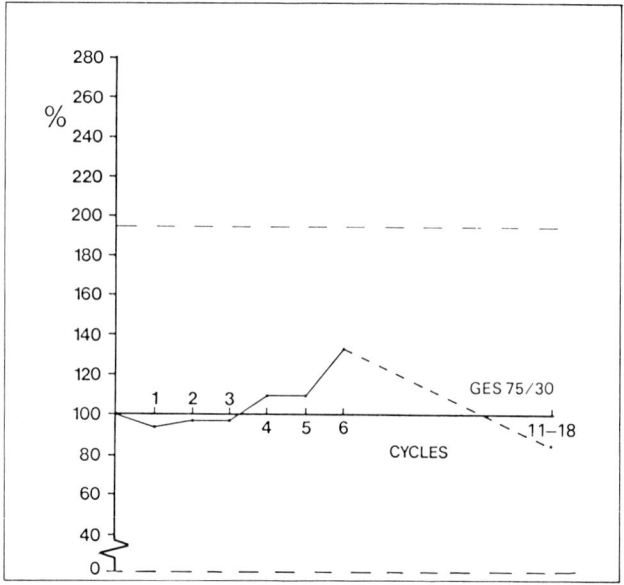

Figure 24   Serum gamma-glutamyl transferase – switch users

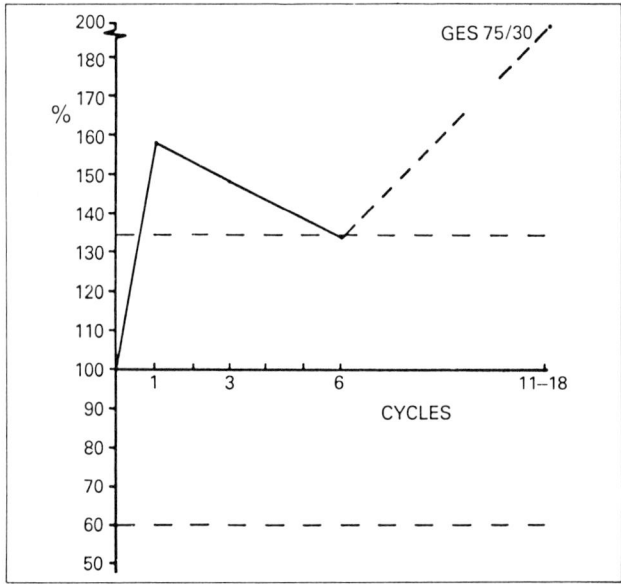

Figure 25   Caeruloplasmin – new users

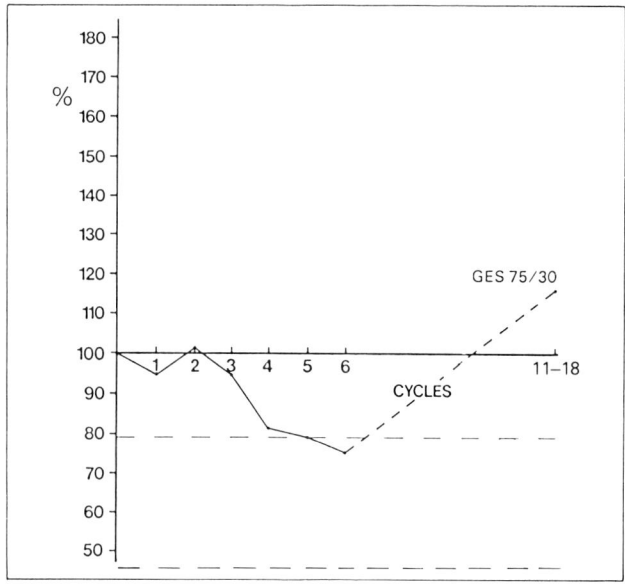

Figure 26   Caeruloplasmin – switch users

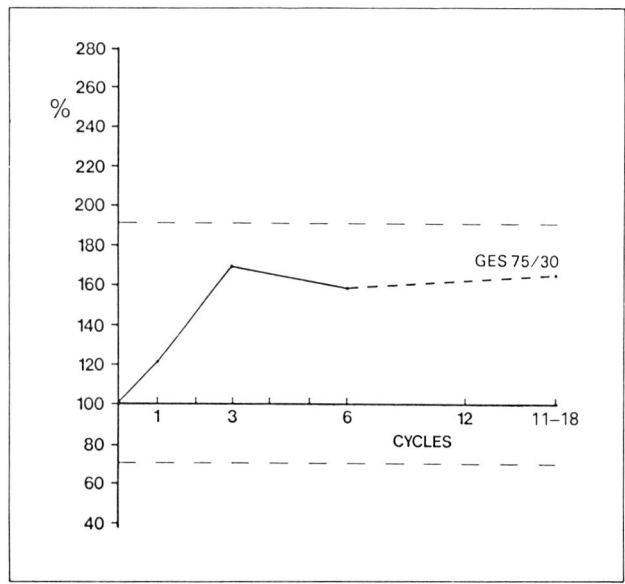

Figure 27   Sex-hormone-binding globulin – new users

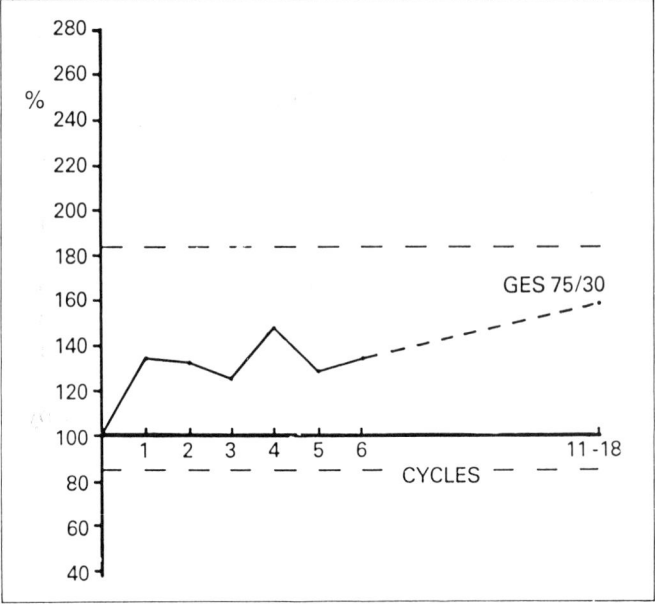

Figure 28   Sex-hormone-binding globulin – switch users

DISCUSSION

Like all the progestogens used in oral contraception, gestodene is a derivative of nortestosterone and has very low androgenic activity. Gestodene's advantage lies in its relatively and absolutely strong progestogenic activity, which permits the use of the uniquely low dose for a combined pill of 75 μg daily.

A simple test of estrogenicity shows that on switching to Femodene from other low-estrogen pills there is, as expected, no change in caeruloplasmin. However, tests that are influenced in opposite directions by the estrogen component and the androgenic activity of the progestogen component – SHBG and lipoproteins – show that androgenic activity is very weak, since SHBG and HDL both rose in switch users, without, of course, any increase in the dose of estrogen. For the same reason, triglycerides and the linked VLDL rose in switch users. However, the initial levels of triglycerides and VLDL were low in the healthy young women studied, and did not rise above about the middle of the normal ranges. Moreover, the more informative ratios of HDL to other lipid fractions were raised by Femodene.

Not only the estrogen component of combined pills, as has long been known, but the progestogen component also, may have an effect on the coagulation system, since Femodene produced a fall in factor X not only to a marked degree in switch users, but even in new users, and although antithrombin III fell slightly in new users there was a marked increase in switch users.

How much clinical significance should we attach to these interim results? Caution should be used in relating the levels after 6 cycles to these shown for long-term use, since the latter were obtained in a cross-sectional study in a different group of women. The differences between pills are small, most of them not statistically significant, and most of the changed levels remain within normal limits.

Nevertheless, without an increase in the estrogen dose, the reduction in progestogen dose made possible by the use of gestodene has provided what are widely held to be desirable changes in HDL and in the coagulation system. Once again, the principle of using the lowest satisfactory dose of each component has been borne out by this new gestodene-containing pill.

Discussion

Editor's note: The following questions and answers have been selected from the manuscript of the discussion. They form a representative cross-section of the discussion but are not a complete record.

QUESTION TO DR ELGER AND DR DÜSTERBERG

I should like to ask Dr Elger and Dr Düsterberg about the endocrinological profile of this new gestodene as regards the very interesting effect on the aldosterone receptors. For the most part, Dr Elger presented data obtained following parenteral administration in animals. Dr Düsterberg, on the other hand, has shown us very interesting metabolites, which are α- and β-hydroxylated in the 3- and 11-positions. For this reason, I wonder whether it would not be worth while for clinicians to see whether this steroid, in its metabolite forms, has different effects on the blood pressure than the classical, older oral contraceptive preparations.

This is purely hypothetical, but I think it is a hypothesis worth looking into.

Dr Elger

Perhaps I should say, first of all, why we work with parenteral administration in the rat experiments. Nortestosterone derivatives have a low bioavailability in rats and a very short half-life, so that daily oral administration only would inhibit ovulation – if at all – in mg doses. Parenteral administration in oily solution, on the other hand, produces pharmacokinetic and pharmacodynamic effects like those observed with oral administration in human beings. Thus, we think that parenteral administration is a better model situation than other alternatives.

As to the anti-aldosterone effect, it must be said that this effect appears at dosage levels which are much higher than those required for contraceptive purposes. The principle is certainly highly interesting, for we may assume that everything which nature does has biological significance. Progesterone has this spectrum of properties, and it is possible that some of the effects which estrogens have on the renin-angiotensin-aldosterone system are compensated by these properties. However, it is extraordinarily difficult to prove this in animal experiments, and it will certainly not be a simple problem to do so in the clinical situation also.

Dr Düsterberg

I would like to say something about the metabolites. In the case of this substance we are in the fortunate position of having elucidated a large number of their molecular structures at this early stage. Still, one should note that only a portion of the dose which was administered led to the formation of these metabolites. We have not yet been able to identify all the metabolites. The hydroxylated metabolites in particular are present in the plasma and the urine as conjugates – i.e., as glucuronides and sulphates – and for this reason they very probably have no endocrine-pharmacological effects. On the other hand, we should follow up this suggestion and test the identified structures pharmacologically.

Professor Kuhl

I would like to make a short comment. If I am recapitulating correctly, gestodene has a stronger binding affinity to the androgen receptor than levonorgestrel, but has a markedly weaker androgenic effect. This is a good example of the care one has to take in making direct correlations between binding constants and clinical effects.

QUESTION TO DR DÜSTERBERG

My question concerns the determination of the bioavailability of gestodene. In your experiments you compared the oral dose with a single intravenous injection. I agree that this is the usual method of determining the bioavailability, but it seems to me that it is not a valid method for most of the steroid compounds. What you really want to do is to compare oral administration with the dose of the new steroid given by intravenous infusion to produce a similar serum concentration-time-curve because, when you compare oral administration with a single i.v. injection, your serum concentration-time-curves are so completely different that it is not really possible to compare them on a valid basis.

Dr Düsterberg

I agree that it is possible to measure the area under the curve more exactly with an infusion than with a single i.v. injection. On the other hand, I believe that we cannot discount the greater technical problems which this method involves. Furthermore, the half-life of gestodene is long enough to allow complete measurement of the area after an i.v. bolus injection as well.

QUESTION TO DR EYONG
I must congratulate Dr Eyong on his very nice paper. However, it is a little bit unclear to me why you chose to start on day 8. Thinking of developing a new contraceptive, why start very late in the cycle?

Dr Eyong
We decided to start on day 8 in order to allow the follicle to develop to about 1 cm size and then see what influence progestogen would exert upon such a follicle. For instance, there was a case where a follicle was 12 mm on day 8 and by day 18 it was reduced to 6 mm. So we saw some inhibition on follicular development and that was more pronounced in group (a) than in group (b).

Dr Lachnit
I think that the final aim of this particular study was *not* to demonstrate the contraceptive efficacy of combined products which would later be developed, but to demonstrate possible differences between the activity of the two progestogens – gestodene and levonorgestrel.

Professor Elstein
Dr Lachnit is absolutely correct. This was a biological study, done in the best biological model – human females – using their uteri. The reason for the day 8 start was that we wanted to be sure that follicular development had been established *before* the progestogen was given.

QUESTION
Did the data Mrs Unger showed us also include the figures which Dr Kirkman presented, or not?

Mrs Unger
The data obtained in England are not included in the study on which I reported.

QUESTION
The preparation containing gestodene had a much lower rate of break-through bleeding than did Microgynon, i.e., 1.8% as compared with 3.1%. Is that statistically significant?

Mrs Unger
Yes, the difference is significant. We have a possible explanation for this fact. Professor Brosens's group has done histological studies on a triphasic preparation whose total hormone content is practically identical with that of Femodene®. This study shows that there were scarcely any sinusoidal vascular changes in the endometrium with

the triphasic preparation which contained gestodene. The team believes that this could be the reason for the excellent cycle control.

QUESTION
Is this new monophasic preparation intended as a successor to Microgynon?

Dr Lachnit
We view Femodene[R] as a further development in the area of monophasic low-dose preparations in general.

Conclusion

M. Elstein

To sum up is difficult. I will try to highlight some of the major points. We have reached a stage of fine tuning of the combined oral contraceptives. We are now in the second decade of Microgynon, which is still a very well tolerated and well accepted oral contraceptive, just as the norethisterone-combined preparations are for some women. There is a considerable background of good contraceptives that have been well tolerated.

We are now moving into a new phase of hormonal contraception and the most important aspect of this is the reduction in their dosage. This has already occurred with the triphasics with less change in metabolic parameters. And now there is gestodene. Biochemically it is a very effective progestogen. The basic scientific data indicated that very clearly, and it is supported by the data on the human female. The combined preparations discussed here have half the dose of progestogen compared with other monophasic formulations and that is a very significant drop in dosage. Biologically it has very potent suppressing action of the gonadotropins, and allows more receptors to be available. It also affects excellent genital tract action as manifested by the cervical mucus changes, giving an ancillary contraceptive mechanism.

As far as the clinical side is concerned, in spite of the low dosage there is excellent cycle control, even better than that of the existing formulations at the higher dosage. The bleeding pattern seems to stabilize itself more quickly, but clearly further data are required to support this. Metabolically, it is interesting that there are these little changes above and below the mean and what is more important for all to see, that all these changes are within the normal range. That is the relevant message, that this is a very fine adjustment of dose.

The overall pattern of this progestogen is that it induces the least change. That is the important aspect because the good Lord made women to function in the way they are, without changing them. Therefore we should try to induce a contraceptive effect without changing the woman's biochemistry significantly. I am not at all impressed when statements are made that the woman's biochemistry has been altered in a favourable way. Surely the object for a contraceptive prescription should be the least change in her bodily function over and above the anti-fertility effect. Gestodene causes lesser changes in metabolic parameters such as lipoproteins, carbohydrate function and hemostatic factors. Long-term epidemiological studies will reveal the significance of this.

For the future, further adjustments in dosage and formulation will be directed to even greater acceptability and comfort to the acceptors of the preparations containing this progestogen. The estrogenic manifestations of this combination are interesting and perhaps a lower estrogen dosage may be possible in the near future which would be even more favourable and to the benefit of the women concerned.

Index